KNOWING WHAT WORKS IN HEALTH CARE

A ROADMAP FOR THE NATION

Committee on Reviewing Evidence to Identify
Highly Effective Clinical Services
Board on Health Care Services

Jill Eden, Ben Wheatley, Barbara McNeil, and Harold Sox, *Editors*

INSTITUTE OF MEDICINE
OF THE NATIONAL ACADEMIES

THE NATIONAL ACADEMIES PRESS
Washington, D.C.
www.nap.edu

THE NATIONAL ACADEMIES PRESS   500 Fifth Street, N.W.   Washington, DC 20001

NOTICE: The project that is the subject of this report was approved by the Governing Board of the National Research Council, whose members are drawn from the councils of the National Academy of Sciences, the National Academy of Engineering, and the Institute of Medicine. The members of the committee responsible for the report were chosen for their special competences and with regard for appropriate balance.

This study was supported by Grant No. 56822 between the National Academy of Sciences and the Robert Wood Johnson Foundation. Any opinions, findings, conclusions, or recommendations expressed in this publication are those of the author(s) and do not necessarily reflect the view of the organizations or agencies that provided support for this project.

Library of Congress Cataloging-in-Publication Data

Knowing what works in health care : a roadmap for the nation / Committee on Reviewing Evidence to Identify Highly Effective Clinical Services, Board on Health Care Services ; Jill Eden ... [et al.], editors.
        p. ; cm.
    Includes bibliographical references.
    ISBN 978-0-309-11356-4 (hardcover)
    1. Medical care--Standards—United States. 2. Medical care—United States—Quality control. 3. Evidence-based medicine—United States. I. Eden, Jill. II. Institute of Medicine (U.S.). Committee on Reviewing Evidence to Identify Highly Effective Clinical Services.
    [DNLM: 1. Quality Assurance, Health Care—standards—United States. 2. Evidence-Based Medicine—standards—United States. 3. Organizational Innovation—United States. 4. Practice Guidelines as Topic—standards—United States. W 84 AA1 K73 2008]
    RA399.A3K56 2008
    362.1--dc22
                                                2008008578

Additional copies of this report are available from the National Academies Press, 500 Fifth Street, N.W., Lockbox 285, Washington, DC 20055; (800) 624-6242 or (202) 334-3313 (in the Washington metropolitan area); Internet, http://www.nap.edu.

For more information about the Institute of Medicine, visit the IOM home page at: **www.iom.edu.**

The serpent has been a symbol of long life, healing, and knowledge among almost all cultures and religions since the beginning of recorded history. The serpent adopted as a logotype by the Institute of Medicine is a relief carving from ancient Greece, now held by the Staatliche Museen in Berlin.

Suggested citation: Institute of Medicine (IOM). 2008. *Knowing what works in health care: A roadmap for the nation.* Washington, DC: The National Academies Press.

"Knowing is not enough; we must apply.
Willing is not enough; we must do."
—Goethe

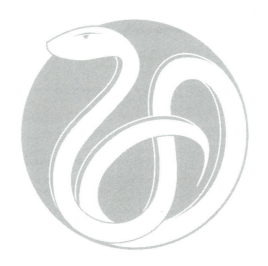

INSTITUTE OF MEDICINE
OF THE NATIONAL ACADEMIES

Advising the Nation. Improving Health.

THE NATIONAL ACADEMIES
Advisers to the Nation on Science, Engineering, and Medicine

The **National Academy of Sciences** is a private, nonprofit, self-perpetuating society of distinguished scholars engaged in scientific and engineering research, dedicated to the furtherance of science and technology and to their use for the general welfare. Upon the authority of the charter granted to it by the Congress in 1863, the Academy has a mandate that requires it to advise the federal government on scientific and technical matters. Dr. Ralph J. Cicerone is president of the National Academy of Sciences.

The **National Academy of Engineering** was established in 1964, under the charter of the National Academy of Sciences, as a parallel organization of outstanding engineers. It is autonomous in its administration and in the selection of its members, sharing with the National Academy of Sciences the responsibility for advising the federal government. The National Academy of Engineering also sponsors engineering programs aimed at meeting national needs, encourages education and research, and recognizes the superior achievements of engineers. Dr. Charles M. Vest is president of the National Academy of Engineering.

The **Institute of Medicine** was established in 1970 by the National Academy of Sciences to secure the services of eminent members of appropriate professions in the examination of policy matters pertaining to the health of the public. The Institute acts under the responsibility given to the National Academy of Sciences by its congressional charter to be an adviser to the federal government and, upon its own initiative, to identify issues of medical care, research, and education. Dr. Harvey V. Fineberg is president of the Institute of Medicine.

The **National Research Council** was organized by the National Academy of Sciences in 1916 to associate the broad community of science and technology with the Academy's purposes of furthering knowledge and advising the federal government. Functioning in accordance with general policies determined by the Academy, the Council has become the principal operating agency of both the National Academy of Sciences and the National Academy of Engineering in providing services to the government, the public, and the scientific and engineering communities. The Council is administered jointly by both Academies and the Institute of Medicine. Dr. Ralph J. Cicerone and Dr. Charles M. Vest are chair and vice chair, respectively, of the National Research Council.

www.national-academies.org

Reviewers

This report has been reviewed in draft form by individuals chosen for their diverse perspectives and technical expertise, in accordance with procedures approved by the National Research Council's (NRC's) Report Review Committee. The purpose of this independent review is to provide candid and critical comments that will assist the institution in making its published report as sound as possible and to ensure that the report meets institutional standards for objectivity, evidence, and responsiveness to the study charge. The review comments and draft manuscript remain confidential to protect the integrity of the deliberative process. We wish to thank the following individuals for their review of this report:

STEVEN FINDLAY, Consumers Union
R. BRIAN HAYNES, Department of Clinical Epidemiology and
    Biostatistics, McMaster University
KATHLEEN McCORMICK, SAIC: Health Solutions
CYNTHIA MULROW, Annals of Internal Medicine
MARY O'NEIL MUNDINGER, School of Nursing, Columbia
    University
PETER NEUMANN, Center for the Evaluation of Value & Risk in
    Health, Tufts-New England Medical Center
SANDRA SCHNEIDER, Department of Emergency Medicine,
    University of Rochester
CARY S. SENNETT, American Board of Internal Medicine
PAUL SHEKELLE, Southern California Evidence-Based Practice
    Center at The RAND Corporation

SHOSHANNA SOFAER, School of Public Affairs, Baruch College
STEVEN TEUTSCH, Outcomes Research & Management, Merck & Co., Inc.
PAUL WALLACE, Health and Productivity Management Programs and The Care Management Institute and KP-Healthy Solutions, The Permanente Federation, Kaiser Permanente

Although the reviewers listed above have provided many constructive comments and suggestions, they were not asked to endorse the conclusions or recommendations nor did they see the final draft of the report before its release. The review of this report was overseen by **SHELDON GREENFIELD,** Center for Health Policy Research, University of California, Irvine, and **JOHANNA T. DWYER,** Tufts University School of Medicine & Friedman School of Nutrition Science, Tufts-New England Medical Center. Appointed by the NRC and the Institute of Medicine, they were responsible for making certain that an independent examination of this report was carried out in accordance with institutional procedures and that all review comments were carefully considered. Responsibility for the final content of this report rests entirely with the authoring committee and the institution.

Preface

The United States has the most expensive health care in the world by a large margin. However, by many measures of the health of the public, the United States ranks well down the list of nations. How can we understand this paradox? The wide regional variation in practice style implies that our knowledge about effective health care is weak enough to support a wide range of accepted practice. Since health care outcomes are the same in high- and low-intensity regions, a lean style of practice is safe and an extravagant style is wasteful.

The regional variation story offers further hints about a way out of this problem. Variation is very low for some practices (e.g., coronary bypass surgery or surgery for fractured hip), which implies secure knowledge and strong consensus. Regional variation is very high for other practices (e.g., MRI and CT scans, ICU admissions in the last six months of life, referral to a specialist), which implies weak knowledge and no consensus. Taken as a whole, the evidence implies that better knowledge could lead to a stronger consensus, less regional variation, and probably lower costs. In short, we need better knowledge of which health care services are the most effective and which patients are most likely to benefit from them.

Concern about the cost of health care has grown in the past 20 years, and organizations that pay for health care have sought to obtain trust-worthy information about what works in the practice of medicine. Payers, government, health care delivery systems, and professional organizations have taken the lead in efforts to develop standards of care. The result has been movement in the right direction, but also chaos. The positive features of these efforts include steady movement away from sole reliance on expert opinion and toward scientific, systematic reviews of the pertinent medical literature and increasing recognition that we need a common language for rating the evidence. The negative features are those inherent in a pluralistic, uncoordinated health care system: large-scale duplication of effort, wide variation in process, far too little attention to avoiding conflict of interest, and lack of standards. We must build on the developing strengths of the present system as we correct these problems.

In the past several years, people have begun to talk about imposing order on the system for identifying effective health services. Many people—ranging from health care experts to payers to presidential candidates—have proposed a national organization to identify the most effective health care services. Somewhat in advance of these proposals, the Robert Wood Johnson Foundation asked the Institute of Medicine (IOM) to convene a committee to recommend methods to identify highly effective health care services. The confluence of these two developments creates what the committee hopes will be a useful contribution to the emerging consensus that the United States needs a more systematic approach to evaluating the evidence for clinical effectiveness.

The IOM committee has focused on specifying the principles underlying the methods to accomplish three crucial tasks for a national system for identifying highly effective health services: priority setting, evidence review, and development of recommendations. We believe that this report would serve to guide an organization tasked with putting a working system into place. In effect, it would be the starting point for a detailed manual of operations for a new organization. In accord with its charge, the committee did not make recommendations about funding for clinical effectiveness research or the institutional home of a national organization for clinical effectiveness.

We expect considerable debate about the committee's recommendation about the structure of this organization. The committee proposes a hybrid structure that exerts control over the processes of setting priorities for which services to evaluate and conducting evidence reviews on the high-priority topics. For the last step—the development of clinical recommendations—the committee proposes to use the nation's existing capacity for developing practice guidelines and insurance coverage policy. The committee proposes standards to guide these organizations in making clinical recommendations and strongly recommends that organizations preferentially use recommendations that are developed according to these standards. For all three tasks, the committee has specific recommendations about minimizing bias due to conflict of interest.

The committee wrote this report for several audiences. One will decide how to allocate resources for a national clinical effectiveness assessment system. Among these are members of the U.S. Congress and private organizations that would benefit from a national clinical effectiveness assessment program. Another audience consists of the organizations that would use the evidence that the new system would produce: payers, health insurance companies, and health care delivery systems. A third audience is the organizations that develop recommendations that will shape practice measures, practice guidelines, and insurance coverage policy. Finally, we hope that members of the general public—the ultimate beneficiaries of the committee's work—will read the report and support efforts to move in the directions proposed in this report.

The IOM chose committee members who—individually and collectively—have the expertise to make credible proposals. Among its members are medical directors of large health insurance companies, health care delivery systems, and companies. The committee also includes physicians with experience in evidence-based guideline programs, experts on extracting evidence from the medical literature, and experienced advocates for the public interest. The breadth of interests represented on the committee is the best guarantee that its recommendations would meet the needs of a diverse community of interest. The committee developed a common vision early in its deliberations, and it speaks with one voice in this report. In a series of workshops, the committee listened to an array of experts who kindly donated their time to help the committee. Above all, the committee had a remarkable group of IOM staff members who supported the committee's efforts and kept the project moving forward. To all, we give thanks.

Barbara J. McNeil, *Chair*
Harold C. Sox, *Vice Chair*

Acknowledgments

The committee and staff are indebted to a number of individuals and organizations for their contributions to this report. The following individuals testified before the committee during public meetings or workshops:

Marilyn Albert, Johns Hopkins University School of Medicine, Division of Cognitive Neuroscience

Naomi Aronson, Blue Cross and Blue Shield Association Technology Evaluation Center

Mary Barton, U.S. Preventive Services Task Force

Barry Berger, Exact Sciences Corporation

Kathy Buto, Johnson & Johnson, Health Policy

Daniel Cain, Cain Brothers

Carolyn Clancy, Agency for Healthcare Research and Quality

Vivian Coates, ECRI Institute

Janet Corrigan, National Quality Forum

Steven Findlay, Consumers Union

Ray Gibbons, American Heart Association

Richard Goldberg, University of North Carolina, Chapel Hill, School of Medicine Division of Hematology & Oncology

Winifred Hayes, Hayes, Inc.

Clarion Johnson, ExxonMobil, Global Medicine and Population Health

Peter Juhn, Johnson & Johnson, Health Policy and Evidence

Michael Maciosek, HealthPartners Foundation

Daniel Martin, Emory University School of Medicine

David Matchar, Duke University Medical School, Center for Clinical
    Health Policy Research
Susan Molchan, Alzheimer's Disease Neuroimaging Initiative,
    National Institute on Aging
Cynthia Mulrow, University of Texas/American College of Physicians
Dennis O'Leary, Joint Commission
Gregory Pawlson, National Committee for Quality Assurance
Stephen Phurrough, Centers for Medicare & Medicaid Services,
    Coverage and Analysis Group
Margaret Piper, Blue Cross and Blue Shield Association Technology
    Evaluation Center
Atiqur Rahman, Food and Drug Administration, Center for Drug
    Evaluation and Research
David Ransohoff, Lineberger Comprehensive Cancer Center,
    University of North Carolina, Chapel Hill
Reginald Sanders, American Society of Retina Specialists
Cary Sennett, AMA-Convened Physician Consortium for Performance
    Improvement
Jean Slutsky, Agency for Healthcare Research and Quality
Arthur Small, Genentech
Earl Steinberg, Resolution Health
Sean Tunis, Center for Medical Technology Policy
Jim Weinstein, Dartmouth Hitchcock Medical Center

We also extend special thanks to the following individuals who were essential sources of information, generously giving their time and knowledge
to further the committee's efforts. Michael A. Stoto, Georgetown University,
and Perry W. Payne, Jr., George Washington University, drafted important
background papers. Kerry Kemp provided valuable editorial assistance.
The following individuals answered many inquiries and were patient with
staff's many requests for information: Mary Barton, U.S. Preventive Ser-
vices Task Force; Kristen K. Bronner, The Dartmouth Atlas; Vivian Coates,
ECRI Institute; Winifred Hayes and Wendy Schneider, Hayes, Inc.; Mark
Helfand, Oregon Health & Science University, Evidence-based Practice
Center; Marguerite Koster, Medical Technology Assessment & Guidelines,
Kaiser Permanente Southern California; Alison S. Little, Oregon Health &
Science University, Drug Effectiveness Review Project; Robert McDonough,
Technology Assessment and Clinical Guidelines, Aetna/US Healthcare; Peter
Neumann and Jenny Palmer, Tufts-New England Medical Center, Center
for the Evaluation of Value and Risk in Health; Chuck Phelps, University
of Rochester; Richard N. Shiffman, Yale University Center for Medical

Informatics; Jean Slutsky, AHRQ Effective Health Care Program; and Gail Wilensky, Project Hope.

Funding for this study was provided by the Robert Wood Johnson Foundation (RWJF). The committee appreciates the opportunity and support extended by RWJF for the development of this report.

Finally, many within the IOM were helpful to the study staff. The staff would especially like to thank Lara Andersen, Clyde Behney, Michelle Bruno, Evalyne Bryant-Ward, Abbey Burchman, Bethany Hardy, Bronwyn Schrecker Jamrok, William McLeod, and Janice Mehler.

Contents

List of Boxes, Figures, and Tables

Chapter 5

Chapter 6

Summary[1]

In the early 21st century, despite unprecedented advances in biomedical knowledge and the highest per capita health care expenditures in the world, the quality and outcomes of health care vary dramatically across the United States. The economic burden of health spending is weakening American industry's competitive edge and consumers are increasingly asked to take on a greater share of the burden. Consumer-directed health care is viewed by some as a means to rationalize what most agree is a health system plagued by overuse, underuse, and misuse. Yet even the most sophisticated health consumer struggles to learn which care is appropriate for his or her circumstance.

It is in this context that the Robert Wood Johnson Foundation asked the Institute of Medicine (IOM) to examine how the nation uses scientific evidence to identify highly effective clinical services. The IOM appointed the Committee on Reviewing Evidence to Identify Highly Effective Clinical Services in June 2006 to respond to the foundation's request (Box S-1). The committee was charged with recommending a sustainable, replicable approach to identifying effective clinical services. Ultimately, the committee concluded that the nation must significantly expand its capacity to use scientific evidence to assess "what works" in health care. This report recommends an organizational framework for a national clinical effectiveness assessment program, referred to throughout as "the Program." The Program's mission would be to optimize the use of evidence to identify effective health

---

[1]This summary does not include references. Citations for the findings presented in the summary appear in the subsequent chapters.

1

BOX S-1
Charge to the IOM Committee

The committee was charged with recommending a sustainable, replicable approach to identifying and evaluating the clinical services that have the highest potential effectiveness. The charge specified three principal tasks:

(1) To recommend an approach to identifying highly effective clinical services across the full spectrum of health care services—from prevention, diagnosis, treatment, and rehabilitation, to end-of-life care and palliation
(2) To recommend a process to evaluate and report on evidence on clinical effectiveness
(3) To recommend an organizational framework for using evidence reports to develop recommendations on appropriate clinical applications for specified populations

---

services. Three functions would be central to this mission: setting priorities for evidence assessment, assessing evidence (systematic review), and developing (or endorsing) standards for trusted clinical practice guidelines.

CONCEPTUAL FRAMEWORK

The committee based its work on the central premise that decisions about the care of individual patients should be based on the conscientious, explicit, and judicious use of current best evidence. This means that individual clinical expertise should be integrated with the best information from scientifically based, systematic research and applied in light of the patient's values and circumstances. Centering decision making on the patient is integral to improving the quality of health care and is also imperative if consumers are to take an active role in making informed health care decisions based on known risks and benefits. This report also recognizes that health care resources are finite. Thus, setting priorities for systematic assessment of scientific evidence is essential.

The era of physician as sole health care decision maker is long past. In today's world, health care decisions are made by multiple people, individually or in collaboration, in multiple contexts for multiple purposes. The decision maker is likely to be the consumer choosing among health plans, patients or patients' caregivers making treatment choices, payers or employers making health coverage and reimbursement decisions, professional medical societies developing practice guidelines or clinical recommendations, regulatory agencies assessing new drugs or devices, or public programs developing population-based health interventions. Every decision maker needs credible, unbiased, and understandable evidence on the effectiveness of health interventions and services.

What constitutes evidence that a health service is effective? Scientists view evidence of effectiveness as knowledge that is explicit, systematic, and replicable. However, patients, clinicians, payers, and other decision makers, often have a different, more contextual perspective on what constitutes evidence of effectiveness. Decision makers consider the scientific evidence as demonstrating what works under ideal circumstances, but of necessity are also interested in "real world" circumstances. Patient factors such as comorbidities, underlying risk, adherence to therapies, disease stage and severity, health insurance coverage, and demographics; intervention factors such as care setting, level of training, and timing and quality of intervention; and other factors can affect the applicability of the results of an individual study to a particular clinical decision or circumstance. There cannot be a single study that covers all populations, intervention approaches, and settings related to a clinical question. Systematic reviews of multiple high-quality studies have the advantage of providing summaries of the available research, which typically covers many different circumstances, and providing a snapshot of where more research is needed.

The conceptual context for this study is the continuum that begins with research evidence, then moves to systematic review of the overall body of evidence, and then to the interpretation of the strength of the overall evidence for developing credible, clinical practice guidelines (Figure S-1). Individual studies rarely provide definitive answers to clinical effectiveness questions. A "systematic review" is a scientific investigation that focuses on a specific question and uses explicit, preplanned scientific methods to identify, select, assess, and summarize similar but separate studies. Systematic reviews are critical to developing agendas for further research because they reveal where evidence is insufficient and additional research is needed. Moreover, a systematic review of studies on clinical effectiveness provides an essential bridge between the body of research evidence and the development of clinical guidance.

AN IMPERATIVE FOR CHANGE

The committee believes that unbiased, reliable information about what works in health care is essential to addressing several persistent health policy challenges (described below).

- *Constraining health care costs.* A significant proportion of health care costs are directed to care that has not been shown to be effective and may actually be harmful.

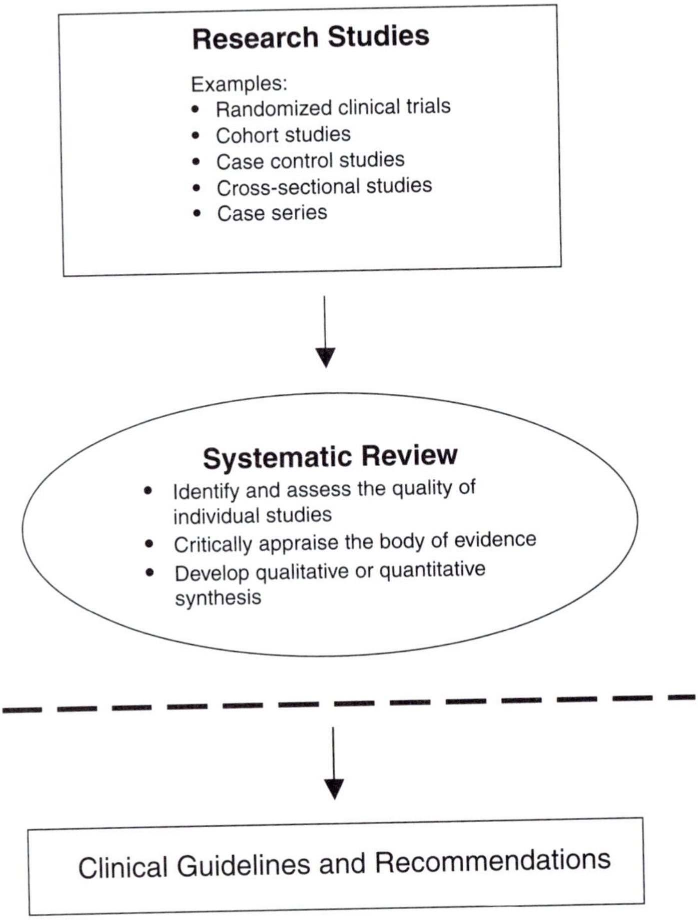

Research Studies

Examples:
- Randomized clinical trials
- Cohort studies
- Case control studies
- Cross-sectional studies
- Case series

Systematic Review
- Identify and assess the quality of individual studies
- Critically appraise the body of evidence
- Develop qualitative or quantitative synthesis

Clinical Guidelines and Recommendations

FIGURE S-1 Continuum from research studies to systematic review to development of clinical guidelines and recommendations.

NOTE: The dashed line is the theoretical dividing line between the systematic review of the research literature and its application to clinical decision making, including the development of clinical guidelines and recommendations. Below the dashed line, decision makers and developers of clinical recommendations interpret the findings of systematic reviews to decide which patients, health care settings, or other circumstances they relate to.

SOURCE: Adapted from West, S., V. King, T. Carey, K. Lohr, N. McCoy, S. Sutton, and L. Lux. 2002. *Systems to rate the strength of scientific evidence. Evidence Report/Technology Assessment No. 47. (Prepared by the Research Triangle Institute-University of North Carolina Evidence-based Practice Center under Contract No. 290-97-0011). AHRQ Publication No. 02-E016.* Rockville, MD: Agency for Healthcare Research and Quality.

- *Reducing geographic variation in the use of health care services.* Variations in treatment patterns often reflect deviations from accepted care standards or uncertainty and disagreement regarding what those standards should be. Uncertainties about what works and for whom means patients cannot always be assured that they will receive the best, most effective care.
- *Improving quality.* To promote quality health care, scientific knowledge should be employed, but the evidence base needed to support effective care is in many instances lacking.
- *Consumer-directed health care.* Many policy makers believe in empowering consumers and patients to be prudent managers of their own health and health care. However, consumers need information on the effectiveness, risks, and benefits of alternative treatments if they are to search for and obtain high-value treatments. The current dearth of such information is a substantial obstacle to consumer empowerment.
- *Making health coverage decisions.* Private and public health plans are struggling with an almost daily challenge of learning how their covered populations might benefit—or be harmed by—newly available health services.

LIMITATIONS IN THE STATUS QUO

There is ample evidence that, under the status quo, there are critical limitations in how the United States identifies and uses evidence on clinical effectiveness, particularly with respect to three interrelated processes: (1) setting priorities for evidence assessment; (2) assessing evidence through systematic reviews; and (3) developing trusted clinical practice guidelines.

Setting Priorities for Evidence Assessment

If we are to resolve current deficiencies in how the nation uses scientific evidence to identify the most effective clinical services, there must be a process for identifying the most important topics in order to preserve resources for evidence assessment itself. Most health technology assessment programs have an organized process for determining which topics merit comprehensive study. But currently no one agency or organization in the United States assumes a broad, national perspective on new as well as established health interventions across all populations—children as well as elderly persons, women as well as men, and including ethnic and racial minorities.

The basic elements of a priority setting process include: identifying potential topics; selecting the priority criteria; reducing the initial list of nominated topics to a smaller set to be pursued; and choosing the final priority topics. Some approaches also incorporate quantitative methods that involve collecting data to weigh priorities, assigning scores for each criterion to each topic, and calculating priority scores for each topic to produce a ranked priority list. The process is typically conducted by a committee or advisory group that reviews and chooses the topics that will be funded. It may employ a formal method, such as the Delphi technique, to systematically develop the high-priority list.

The committee could not find any systematic assessments of the comparative strengths and weaknesses of different approaches to setting priorities, including whether complex, quantitative, and resource-intensive methods are more effective than less rigorous approaches. Many organizations report using the same general criteria to gauge the potential impact that an evidence assessment might have on clinical care and patient outcomes. These include burden of disease (rates of disability, morbidity, or mortality), public controversy, cost (related to the condition, the procedure, in the aggregate), new evidence that might change previously held conclusions (new clinical trial results), adequacy of the existing evidence, and unexplained variation in use of services. How these factors play into final priorities is not apparent.

At present, there is substantial unnecessary duplication in reviews of new and emerging technologies. Decision makers, especially in health plans and health systems, often need to learn quickly about new and emerging technologies and what is known and not known about effectiveness. Patients and providers want information on new health services as soon as they become available, often because manufacturers are pressing them to adopt a product or because consumers have been exposed to direct-to-consumer advertising and want answers from their physician. Yet, almost by definition, sufficient objective information about new and emerging technologies is seldom available. New and emerging technologies may require a different priority setting process—including separate criteria—than other topics with more substantive evidence.

Systematic Reviews Are the Central Link Between Evidence and Clinical Decision Making

Systematic reviews of evidence on the effectiveness of health services provide a central link between the generation of research and clinical decision making. Individual studies rarely provide definitive answers to clinical effectiveness questions. If conducted properly, the systematic review should make obvious the gap between what is known about the effectiveness of a particular service and what clinicians and patients want to know. As such, systematic reviews are also critical to developing the agenda for further primary research because they reveal where evidence is insufficient and new information is needed. Without systematic reviews, researchers may miss promising leads or pursue questions that have been answered already.

Systematic review is itself a science—a new and dynamic science with evolving methods. In medicine, early implementers were trialists who saw the need to summarize data from multiple effectiveness trials, many of them with very small samples. By the late 1980s, systematic reviews were increasingly used to assess the effectiveness of health interventions but research also began to reveal problems in their execution. The methods underlying the reviews were often neither objective nor transparent. The approach to deciding which literature to include and which findings to present was subjective and nonsystematic. Still today, the quality of published reviews is variable and often unreliable.

The core of a systematic review is a concise and transparent synthesis of the results of the included studies. The language of the review should be simple and clear so that it is usable and accessible to decision makers. The synthesis may be purely qualitative, that is, describing study results individually but not combined, or it may be complemented by meta-analysis that combines the individual study results quantitatively and allows statistical inference.

Under the status quo, judging the quality of reviews is often difficult because methods are so poorly documented. Reviews rely on many disparate grading schemes and evidence hierarchies that are often not well understood. Since the underlying rationale for hierarchies is to present study designs in terms of increasing protections against bias, evidence hierarchies have the potential to raise awareness that some forms of evidence are more trustworthy than others. However, hierarchies are often oversimplified and consider just the type of research (e.g., a clinical trial versus an observational study) and not the question being asked. Observational and experimental studies each can provide valid and reliable evidence, but their relative value depends on the clinical question. For example, randomized controlled trials can best answer questions about the efficacy of screening, preventive, and therapeutic interventions while observational studies are generally the most appropriate for answering questions related to prognosis, diagnostic accuracy, incidence, prevalence, and etiology.

The synthesis should collate, describe, and summarize the following key features of the individual studies it reviews that could have a bearing on the findings:

- Characteristics of the patient population, care setting, and type of provider
- Intervention (route, dose, timing, duration)
- Comparison group
- Outcome measures and timing of assessments

- Quality of the evidence (i.e., risk of bias) from individual studies and possible influence on findings. The term "bias" has different meanings depending on the context in which it is used. It may refer to "bias" due to conflicts of interest. "Bias" also refers to statistical bias, i.e., the tendency for a study to produce results that depart systematically from the truth. Statistical biases can lead to under- or over-estimation of the effectiveness of an intervention
- Sample sizes
- Quantitative results and analyses, including examination of whether the study estimates of effect are consistent across studies
- Examination of potential sources of study heterogeneity, if relevant

The synthesis should not include recommendations. If the systematic review is both scientific and transparent, decision makers should be able to interpret the evidence, to know what is not known, and to describe the extent to which the evidence is applicable to clinical practice and particular subgroups of patients. Making evidence-based decisions—such as when a guideline developer recommends what should and should not be done in specific clinical circumstances—is a distinct and separate process from systematic review.

It is not known how many researchers in the United States are adequately trained and qualified to conduct systematic reviews on the effectiveness of health services.

Developing Evidence-Based Clinical Practice Guidelines

The development of clinical guidelines in the United States today is highly decentralized and involves many public and private organizations—medical professional societies, patient advocacy groups, payers, government agencies, and others. The National Guideline Clearinghouse (NGC) maintained by the Agency for Healthcare Research and Quality includes clinical guidelines from about 360 different organizations. The U.S. Preventive Services Task Force produces recommendations for preventive services that are widely considered to offer a gold standard for the process of guideline development. International organizations also produce clinical guidelines that are available in the United States.

One of the challenges inherent in having a highly decentralized, pluralistic process for developing clinical guidelines is that multiple groups will produce guidelines in the same clinical topic area. Currently, for example, the NGC contains 471 guidelines relating to the topic of hypertension and 276 guidelines related to stroke. Despite the abundance of clinical guidance for some topics, there is little clinical guidance on other important topics.

The translation of evidence into recommendations is not straightforward. Although guideline developers have adopted several strategies to improve the reliability and trustworthiness of the information they provide, it is not yet possible to say that the development of clinical guidelines is based on a scientifically validated process. The key challenges stem from the fact that guideline development frequently forces organizations to go beyond available evidence to make practical recommendations for use in everyday practice. Given the gaps in the evidence base that frequently exist and the variable quality of the information that is available, some observers have suggested that one criterion of an effective guideline process is to have two separate grading systems: one for the quality of evidence and another for the recommendations themselves. Even when there is substantial consensus about the existing scientific evidence, there may be different interpretations about what the evidence means for clinical practice. Different interpretations can be due, for example, to conflicting viewpoints about which outcomes are the most important or which course of action is appropriate given that evidence is imperfect.

RECOMMENDATIONS

The committee recommends the development of a national clinical effectiveness assessment program to facilitate the development of standards and processes that yield credible, unbiased, and understandable syntheses of the available evidence on clinical effectiveness for patients, individual clinicians, health plans, purchasers, specialty societies, and others. The committee hopes that the nation now has the will to address the urgent need to bolster the U.S. health system with a foundation built on research evidence and scientific methods.

The committee recommends a single entity be established to help determine what works in health care. Box S-2 lists all the recommendations presented in this report. Each recommendation is elaborated on in its respective chapter with a rationale and strategies for implementation.

Recommendation: Congress should direct the secretary of the U.S. Department of Health and Human Services to designate a single entity (the Program) with authority, overarching responsibility, sustained resources, and adequate capacity to ensure production of credible, unbiased information about what is known and not known about clinical effectiveness. The Program should

- **set priorities for, fund, and manage systematic reviews of clinical effectiveness and related topics;**
- **develop a common language and standards for conducting system-**

BOX S-2
Recommendations

Building a Foundation (Chapter 6)

Congress should direct the secretary of the U.S. Department of Health and Human Services to designate a single entity (the Program) with authority, overarching responsibility, sustained resources, and adequate capacity to ensure production of credible, unbiased information about what is known and not known about clinical effectiveness. The Program should

- set priorities for, fund, and manage systematic reviews of clinical effectiveness and related topics;
- develop a common language and standards for conducting systematic reviews of the evidence and for generating clinical guidelines and recommendations;
- provide a forum for addressing conflicting guidelines and recommendations; and
- prepare an annual report to Congress.

The secretary of Health and Human Services should appoint a Clinical Effectiveness Advisory Board to oversee the Program. Its membership should be constituted to minimize bias due to conflict of interest and should include representation of diverse public and private sector expertise and interests.

The Program should develop standards to minimize bias due to conflicts of interest for priority setting, evidence assessment, and recommendations development.

Setting Priorities (Chapter 3)

The Program should appoint a standing Priority Setting Advisory Committee (PSAC) to identify high-priority topics for systematic reviews of clinical effectiveness.

- The priority setting process should be open, transparent, efficient, and timely.
- Priorities should reflect the potential for evidence-based practice to improve

---

atic reviews of the evidence and for generating clinical guidelines and recommendations;

- provide a forum for addressing conflicting guidelines and recommendations; and
- prepare an annual report to Congress.

The committee further recommends that an advisory board be appointed to oversee the Program, and that the Program develop (or endorse) standards to minimize bias.

Recommendation: The secretary of Health and Human Services should appoint a Clinical Effectiveness Advisory Board to oversee the Pro-

health outcomes across the life span, reduce the burden of disease and health disparities, and eliminate undesirable variation.
- Priorities should also consider economic factors, such as the costs of treatment and the economic burden of disease.
- The membership of the PSAC should include a broad mix of expertise and interests and be chosen to minimize committee bias due to conflicts of interest.

Systematic Reviews (Chapter 4)

The Program should develop evidence-based methodologic standards for systematic reviews, including a common language for characterizing the strength of evidence. The Program should fund reviewers only if they commit to and consistently meet these standards.

- The Program should invest in advancing the scientific methods underlying the conduct of systematic reviews and, when appropriate, update the standards for the reviews it funds.

The Program should assess the capacity of the research workforce to meet the Program's needs, and, if deemed appropriate, it should expand training opportunities in systematic review and comparative effectiveness research methods.

Developing Trusted Guidelines (Chapter 5)

Groups developing clinical guidelines or recommendations should use the Program's standards, document their adherence to the standards, and make this documentation publicly available.

To minimize bias due to conflicts of interest, panels should include a balance of competing interests and diverse stakeholders, publish conflict of interest disclosures, and prohibit voting by members with material conflicts.

Providers, public and private payers, purchasers, accrediting organizations, performance measurement groups, patients, consumers, and others should preferentially use clinical recommendations developed according to the Program standards.

gram. Its membership should be constituted to minimize bias due to conflict of interest and should include representation of diverse public and private sector expertise and interests.

Recommendation: The Program should develop standards to minimize bias due to conflicts of interest for priority setting, evidence assessment, and recommendations development.

The committee envisions a Program—whether a public entity or a public-private entity—that develops standards and sets priorities and facilitates systematic reviews of priority topics by external organizations. The committee believes that the most pragmatic—and also the most promising—

approach to establishing such a Program is to build on current efforts. In addition, private organizations that currently produce guidelines, such as professional societies and others, treasure their autonomy and would likely oppose efforts to reduce their role. Further, guidelines that have the imprimatur of a respected professional society are able to engender trust in end users. Finally, there are some indications that the quality of these guidelines has improved over time.

The committee wants to ensure that the national Program recommended by the committee is stable over the long term; its output is judged as objective, credible, and without conflict of interest or bias; and its operations are independent of external political pressures. For that reason, the committee recommends that the Program be built on the basis of eight core principles: accountability, consistency, efficiency, feasibility, objectivity, responsiveness, scientific rigor, and transparency (Box S-3).

BOX S-3
Program Principles

Accountability	Parties are directly responsible for meeting standards.
Consistency	Processes are predictable and standardized so as to be readily usable by patients, health professionals, medical societies, payers, and purchasers.
Efficiency	Avoids waste and unnecessary duplication.
Feasibility	Capable of operating in the real world; recognizing political, economic, and social implications.
Objectivity	Evidence-based and without bias, e.g., balanced participation, governance, and standards minimize conflicts of interest and other biases.
Responsiveness	Addresses information needs of decision makers in a timely way. Able to react quickly. Patients and health professionals require real time information for treatment decisions.
Scientific rigor	Methods minimize bias, provide reproducible results, and are completely reported.
Transparency	Methods are explicitly defined, consistently applied, and available for public review so that observers can readily link judgments, decisions, or actions to the data on which they are based.

Recommendations for Setting National Priorities for Systematic Reviews

Setting national priorities for systematic reviews is important because the overall value of the Program will hinge, in part, on how effectively the enterprise determines its priorities. The committee recommends that the Program appoint an independent, free-standing Priority Setting Advisory Committee (PSAC) to develop and implement a priority setting process that will identify those high-priority topics that merit systematic evidence assessment. In contrast to the Clinical Effectiveness Advisory Board, which should provide broad oversight of the Program, the PSAC should be an active advisory body that meets frequently to advise the Program on topics that merit priority systematic review.

Recommendation: The Program should appoint a standing Priority Setting Advisory Committee (PSAC) to identify high-priority topics for systematic reviews of clinical effectiveness.

- The priority setting process should be open, transparent, efficient, and timely.
- Priorities should reflect the potential for evidence-based practice to improve health outcomes across the life span, reduce the burden of disease and health disparities, and eliminate undesirable variation.
- Priorities should also consider economic factors, such as the costs of treatment and the economic burden of disease.
- The membership of the PSAC should include a broad mix of expertise and interests and be chosen to minimize committee bias due to conflicts of interest.

The PSAC should consider a broad range of topics, including, for example, new, emerging, and well-established health services across the full spectrum of health care (e.g., preventive interventions, diagnostic tests, treatments, rehabilitative therapies, and end-of-life care and palliation); community-based interventions such as immunization initiatives or programs to encourage smoking cessation; and research methods and data sources for the analysis of comparative effectiveness.

The highest priorities should focus on the clinical questions of patients and clinicians that have the potential for substantial impact on health outcomes across all ages, burden of disease and health disparities, and undesirable variation in the delivery of health services.

There is limited research evidence to suggest the optimal composition or size of the PSAC. The committee believes it should be sufficiently large to include all of the important stakeholders, but not too large so that it is unwieldy. The membership should mirror the Program's target audience, especially patients and consumers, clinicians, payers, purchasers, guideline developers, and individuals with the appropriate expertise in relevant content areas and technical methods.

The PSAC should cast a wide net to include all stakeholders in an open and transparent topic nomination process. The process should especially cultivate input from end users such as guideline developers, consumers, patients, health professionals, and payers. While the nomination process should not be overly burdensome to potential nominators, there should be standardized methods and information requirements.

Objectivity implies balanced participation, oversight by a governance body, and standards that minimize conflicts of interest and other biases.[2] The PSAC should not be dominated by special interests that can benefit materially or by intellectual biases that might favor one professional specialty over another (e.g., surgery versus medicine, ophthalmology versus optometry).

Using transparent, well-documented, and standard procedures also contribute to perceptions of objectivity. Stakeholders are not likely to trust an unpredictable, opaque process. All deliberations should be open to encourage public participation, public confidence, and ensure a wide variety of perspectives. The PSAC should post key documents on its website, including meeting announcements and decisions concerning priorities, and give time for public comment on documents that support the priority setting process.

Recommendations for Conducting Systematic Reviews

Recommendation: The Program should develop evidence-based, methodologic standards for systematic reviews, including a common language for characterizing the strength of evidence. The Program should fund reviewers only if they commit to and consistently meet these standards.

- The Program should invest in advancing the scientific methods underlying the conduct of systematic reviews and, when appropriate, update the standards for the reviews it funds.

Recommendation: The Program should assess the capacity of the research workforce to meet the Program's needs, and, if deemed appro-

---

[2]The IOM has recently appointed the Committee on Conflict of Interest in Medical Research, Education, and Practice to recommend principles for managing conflicts of interest in the conduct of medical research, development of practice guidelines, and patient care. A final report is expected in 2009 and may provide important guidance to the Program.

priate, it should expand training opportunities in systematic review and comparative effectiveness research methods.

Recommendations for Developing Trusted Clinical Practice Guidelines

Clinical practice guidelines vary widely in their methodological rigor and protection from bias, and the committee recommends that steps be taken to ensure that the information communicated through practice guidelines is trustworthy.

Recommendation: Groups developing clinical guidelines or recommendations should use the Program's standards, document their adherence to the standards, and make this documentation publicly available.

Recommendation: To minimize bias due to conflicts of interest, panels should include a balance of competing interests and diverse stakeholders, publish conflict of interest disclosures, and prohibit voting by members with material conflicts.

Recommendation: Providers, public and private payers, purchasers, accrediting organizations, performance measurement groups, patients, consumers, and others should preferentially use clinical recommendations developed according to the Program standards.

1

Introduction

Abstract: This chapter presents the objectives and context for this report, defines the key concepts used throughout the report, and describes the approach of the Institute of Medicine (IOM) Committee on Reviewing Evidence to Identify Highly Effective Clinical Services to undertaking the study. The committee was charged with recommending an organizational framework for assessing evidence on clinical effectiveness so that consumers, clinicians, professional specialty societies, payers, purchasers, and other decision makers have independent, valid information for making health care decisions. The central premise underlying the report is that decisions about the care of individual patients should be based on the conscientious, explicit, and judicious use of the current best evidence on the effectiveness of clinical services. The conceptual context is the continuum beginning with research evidence, moving to systematic review of the overall body of evidence, and then to interpretation of the strength of the overall evidence for developing evidence-based clinical practice guidelines. The report provides a general blueprint for a national clinical effectiveness assessment program ("the Program") with responsibility for three fundamental processes: (1) setting priorities for evidence assessment, (2) assessing evidence (systematic review), and (3) developing (or endorsing) standards for evidence-based clinical practice guidelines.

In the early 21st century, despite unprecedented advances in biomedical knowledge and the highest per capita health care expenditures in the world, the quality and outcomes of health care vary dramatically across the United States (Fisher and Wennberg, 2003; Fisher et al., 2003a,b; McGlynn et al., 2003). The economic burden of constantly inflating health care spending is weakening American industry's competitive edge and in the global economy, and this burden is increasingly being transferred to consumers as they are held more financially at risk for the health care services that they use (Gabel et al., 2002; U.S. Government Accountability Office, 2006a,b; Webster, 2006). Enabling and incentivizing "consumer choice" is viewed by some as a potential market strategy to rationalize what most agree is a health care system plagued by overuse, underuse, and misuse (Schwartz, 1984; Wennberg, 2004). Yet even the most sophisticated health care consumer struggles to learn which care is appropriate for his or her circumstance and to obtain it at the right time (Berwick, 2003; Rettig et al., 2007; Wennberg, 2002).

With these trends in view, the Robert Wood Johnson Foundation (RWJF) asked the Institute of Medicine (IOM) to address problems in how the nation uses scientific evidence to identify the most effective clinical services. The IOM appointed the Committee on Reviewing Evidence to Identify Highly Effective Clinical Services in June 2006 to respond to RWJF's request and prepare this report. The 16-member committee included experts in clinical research, health care coverage, drug development, health care benefits selection (large employers and other purchasers), health care delivery, clinical guideline development, economics, statistical methods and epidemiology, consumer and patient perspectives, child health, preventive medicine, behavioral health, and ethics. Brief biographies of the committee members appear in Appendix G.

STUDY SCOPE

The committee was charged with recommending a sustainable, replicable approach to identifying and evaluating the clinical services that have the highest potential effectiveness. The charge specified three principal tasks:

(1) To recommend an approach to identifying highly effective clinical services across the full spectrum of health care services—from prevention, diagnosis, treatment, and rehabilitation, to end-of-life care and palliation
(2) To recommend a process to evaluate and report on evidence on clinical effectiveness
(3) To recommend an organizational framework for using evidence reports to develop recommendations on appropriate clinical applications for specified populations

The committee's initial deliberations focused on articulating its charge in a strategic work plan for the 18-month study period. The committee chose to focus on developing an organizational framework for a national clinical effectiveness assessment program, referred to throughout the report as "the Program." The mission of the Program would be to optimize the use of evidence to identify effective health care services. Three functions would be central to this mission: setting priorities for conducting evidence assessments, conducting evidence assessments (systematic review), and developing (or endorsing) standards for trusted clinical practice guidelines. The objective of this report is twofold: first, to examine the scientific rationale for these three functions and, second, to recommend an organizational context for implementing the three functions.

The committee reviewed, and ultimately excluded, a number of topics that might be related to the charge including cost-effectiveness, knowledge transfer and adherence to guidelines, program costs and sources of program funding, placement of the program (e.g., within a governmental or private-sector framework), patient values and preferences, legal issues, and technical methods underlying evidence assessment or guideline development.

The committee explored the relevance of cost and cost-effectiveness analysis (CEA) to the committee's charge over the course of several meetings. The committee decided not to make recommendations about the role of costs in evaluating clinical services for two reasons. First, in the United States, the role of cost in government health policy and coverage decisions, clinical guidelines, and practice measures is unresolved albeit often debated (Congressional Budget Office, 2007; Medicare Payment Advisory Commission, 2007; Wilensky, 2006). Although CEA has been used for decades to estimate the relative value of alternative health interventions, particularly with respect to new prescription medications, most policy makers do not use it explicitly. Many policy makers believe information on cost-effectiveness has the potential to guide more efficient use of health care resources. The committee noted, however, that—regardless of the cost side of the equation—reliable cost-effectiveness analysis depends on high-quality evidence on effectiveness. In fact, the Medicare Payment Advisory Commission has recommended that before policy makers routinely employ CEA for decision making, they must address concerns about CEA methods, including how to assess the effectiveness of health services (Medicare Payment Advisory Commission, 2005). By this reasoning, high-quality comparative effectiveness research is a prerequisite to performing valid cost-effectiveness analyses. Second, RWJF, the sponsor of this study, urged the committee to limit its work to the non-cost issues related to determining the effectiveness of health care services. Following the completion of the IOM study, RWJF intends to fund additional research into how cost affects access to effective health care services (Lumpkin, 2006).

The committee also discussed at length whether the report should delve into issues related to knowledge transfer and adherence to clinical guidelines. Clearly, identifying effective health services is just one step toward ensuring an effective health care system. There is little value to identifying effective services or developing evidence-based practice guidelines, if the knowledge gained does not lead to higher quality health care delivery and improved patient outcomes. However, setting standards for best practices (e.g., through clinical guidelines) differs fundamentally from successfully implementing them through quality improvement projects, which take place at a local level.

STUDY METHODS

The committee deliberated during 5 in-person meetings and 14 telephone conferences between July 2006 and October 2007. As previously noted, during its early discussions, the members of the committee agreed to first develop a strategic work plan for organizing the study. This soon led to a primary focus on three processes deemed integral to identifying effective health care services.

Given the dynamic nature of the issues involved in the study, the committee decided to supplement its planned review of the relevant literature with expert testimony on current issues. It thus convened two public workshops. The first workshop, held in November 2006, focused on evidence generation, evidence synthesis, and evidence assessment of new health care technologies and new applications of existing technologies. The committee heard testimony from various experts, including the developers of health care technologies, government regulators, research scientists, and technology assessors, on their experiences with the use of positron emission tomography scanning for the diagnosis of Alzheimer's disease; pharmacotherapy with bevacizumab (Avastin) and ranibizumab (Lucentis) for age-related macular degeneration; and two technologies related to the early identification and treatment of colorectal cancer; the fecal DNA screening test and an assay to test toxicity for the chemotherapy agent irinotecan.

The second workshop, held in January 2007, focused on organizations that set priorities for developing systematic reviews, clinical practice guidelines, and practice standards. The committee heard testimony from senior representatives of the Agency for Healthcare Research and Quality (AHRQ), the U.S. Preventive Services Task Force (USPSTF), Consumers Union's Best Buy Drugs, the American Heart Association (in collaboration with the American College of Cardiology), the National Quality Forum, the National Committee for Quality Assurance, the Joint Commission, the American Medical Association (AMA)-convened Physician Consortium for Performance Improvement, UnitedHealthcare, the Cochrane Collaboration, the Blue Cross and Blue Shield Association Technology Evaluation Center (an Evidence-based Practice Center), Johnson & Johnson, the ECRI Institute, Genentech, and the Dartmouth-Hitchcock Department of Orthopedic Surgery. In addition to oral testimony, the experts provided written responses to the committee's questions.

Appendix B provides further details on the public workshops.

CONTEXT FOR THIS REPORT

Conceptual Framework

The committee based its work on the central premise that decisions about the care of individual patients should be based on "the conscientious, explicit, and judicious use of current best evidence" (Sackett et al., 1996). This means that individual clinical expertise should be integrated with the best information from scientifically based, systematic research and should be applied in light of the patient's unique values and circumstances (Straus et al., 2005). Centering on the patient is integral to improving the quality of health care (IOM, 2001) and is also imperative if consumers are to take an active role in making informed health care decisions based on known risks and benefits. The committee also recognizes that health care resources are finite. Thus, setting priorities for the systematic assessment of the scientific evidence is essential.

What Is Evidence?

In the everyday sense, "evidence" is considered a collection of facts that ground one's belief that something is true (Dictionary.com, 2007). In searching for evidence that a health care service is highly effective, the notion of what constitutes evidence is more complex. It also depends on one's perspective. In a systematic review of the different views on the nature of evidence, Lomas and colleagues (2005) observed that scientists view evidence as knowledge that is explicit (codified and propositional), systematic (with transparent and explicit methods used to codify the evidence), and replicable. However, outside the research community, decision makers, such as patients, clinicians, health plan managers, and employers, see evidence as being more contextual. For the decision maker, scientific evidence demonstrates what works under ideal circumstances, but it has relevance only when it is adapted to a particular set of circumstances. Someone must interpret the evidence for it to be used to guide clinical decision making.

Who Is a Health Care Decision Maker?

The era of physician as sole health care decision maker is long past. In today's world, health care decisions are made by multiple persons, individually or in collaboration, in multiple contexts for multiple purposes. Decision makers are likely to be the consumer choosing among health plans, patients or the patients' caregivers making treatment choices, payers or employers making health care coverage and reimbursement decisions, professional medical societies developing practice guidelines or clinical recommendations, regulatory agencies assessing new drugs or devices, and public programs developing population-based health interventions. Every decision maker needs credible, unbiased, and understandable evidence on the effectiveness of health care services.

Conceptual Context for the Study

The committee defined the conceptual context for this study as the continuum that begins with research evidence and that then moves to a scientific, systematic review of the overall body of evidence and then to the interpretation of the strength of the overall evidence for the development of trusted clinical practice guidelines (Figure 1-1). The systematic review is an essential element of scientific inquiry into what is known and not known about what works in health care (Glasziou and Haynes, 2005; Helfand, 2005; Mulrow and Lohr, 2001; Steinberg and Luce, 2005). The strength of the evidence depends on the quality of the individual studies that comprise the body of evidence, the combined number of participants and events observed in the relevant studies, the consistency of the findings of the relevant studies, and the magnitude of the observed effects (Higgins and Green, 2006; Khan et al., 2001; West et al., 2002).

What Is an Effective Clinical Service?

The terms "effectiveness" and "clinical effectiveness" refer to the extent to which a specific intervention, procedure, regimen, or service does what it what it is intended to do when it is used under real world circumstances (Cochrane Collaboration, 2005; Last, 2001). Recently, numerous proposals have called for a large expansion in the generation of comparative effectiveness information (BCBSA, 2007a; Congressional Budget Office, 2007; The Health Industry Forum, 2006; IOM, 2007; Medicare Payment Advisory Commission, 2007; Wilensky, 2006). These proposals call for systems to compare the impacts of different options for caring for a medical condition (e.g., prostate cancer) for a defined set of patients (e.g., men at high risk of prostate cancer recurrence). The comparison may be between similar treatments, such as competing prescription medications, or for very different treatment approaches, such as surgery or radiation therapy. Or, the comparison may be between using a specific intervention and its nonuse (sometimes called "watchful waiting"). This report uses the terms

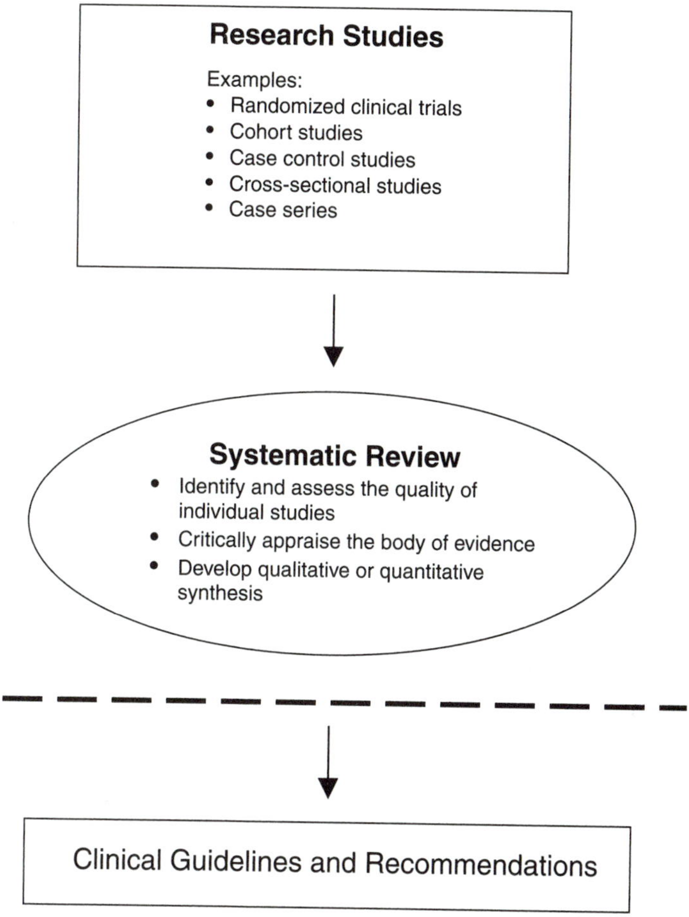

FIGURE 1-1 Continuum from research studies to systematic review to development of clinical guidelines and recommendations.

NOTE: The dashed line is the theoretical dividing line between the systematic review of the research literature and its application to clinical decision making, including the development of clinical guidelines and recommendations. Below the dashed line, decision makers and developers of clinical recommendations interpret the findings of systematic reviews to decide which patients, health care settings, or other circumstances they relate to.

SOURCE: Adapted from *Systems to Rate the Strength of Scientific Evidence* (West et al., 2002).

"effectiveness," "clinical effectiveness," and "comparative effectiveness" interchangeably.

See Box 1-1 for other key terms that are referred to in the report.

Historical Context

This study occurs at a time when there is heightened interest in optimizing U.S. health care through the generation of new knowledge on the

---

BOX 1-1
Selected Terms Used in the Report

Experimental study—A study in which the investigators actively intervene to test a hypothesis. **Controlled trials** are experimental studies in which an experimental group receives the intervention of interest while a comparison group receives no intervention, a placebo, or the standard of care and the outcomes are compared. In a **randomized controlled trial**, the participants are randomly allocated to the experimental group or the comparison group.

Observational or nonexperimental study—A study in which the investigators do not seek to intervene but simply observe the course of events. In **cohort studies**, groups with certain exposures or characteristics are monitored over time to observe an outcome of interest. In **case-control studies**, groups with and without an event or condition are examined to see whether a past exposure or event is more prevalent in one group than in the other. **Cross-sectional studies** determine the prevalence of a condition or an exposure at a specific time or time period. **Case series** describe a group of patients with a characteristic in common, for example, individuals undergoing a new type of surgery or the users of a new device.

Systematic review—A systematic review is a scientific investigation that focuses on a specific question and that uses explicit, preplanned scientific methods to identify, select, assess, and summarize the findings of similar but separate studies. It may or may not include a quantitative synthesis of the results from separate studies (meta-analysis). In this report, the term "systematic review" is used to encompass reviews that incorporate meta-analyses as well as reviews that present the study descriptively rather than inferentially.

Meta-analysis—The process of using statistical methods to combine quantitatively the results of similar studies in an attempt to allow inferences to be made from the sample of studies and applied to the population of interest.

Technology assessment—An assessment of the effectiveness of medical technologies that uses either single studies or systematic reviews.

SOURCES: Cochrane Collaboration (2005); Haynes et al. (2006); Last (2001); West et al. (2002).

effectiveness of health care services. As noted earlier, numerous stakeholders, policy makers, and government entities have proposed substantial new investment in comparative effectiveness research (America's Health Insurance Plans, 2007; BCBSA, 2007a; IOM, 2007; Medicare Payment Advisory Commission, 2007; Wilensky, 2006). These calls for the generation of evidence underscore the urgency of the concern that the nation's health care decision makers be able to discern which evidence is valid, for whom, and under what circumstances. Marked increases in the evidence base for health care decision making will inevitably bring a concomitant need for an increased capability for the synthesis and the interpretation of the evidence.

The recent efforts to expand comparative effectiveness research follow more than four decades of progress and setbacks in this area. Overall, there have been significant gains in the science of effectiveness research, from the adoption of randomized controlled trials in the 1960s to the introduction of technology assessment in the 1970s, the methodological advances of the 1980s, and the creation of the Cochrane Collaboration in the 1990s (Box 1-2). Along the way, various government entities and private organizations have been launched to perform or be responsible for clinical effectiveness research. Many of these initiatives have faltered because of inadequate funding or political conflicts with vested interests (Gray, 1992; Gray et al., 2003). This committee hopes that the nation now has the will to address the urgent need to bolster the U.S. health care system with a foundation built on research evidence and scientific methods.

ORIENTATION TO THE ORGANIZATION OF THE REPORT

This report provides a general blueprint for a national clinical effectiveness assessment program ("the Program"). The overall intent is to outline key Program functions and to recommend an overarching Program infrastructure. The following section describes the organization of the report and the objective of each chapter.

Chapter Objectives

This introductory chapter has described the objectives and context for this report, including the conceptual framework, key terminology, historical context, and methods used to perform the study. The subsequent chapters sequentially outline the building blocks of the Program, i.e., priority setting, assessing evidence (systematic review), and developing (or endorsing) standards for clinical practice guidelines. The final chapter explores how best to organize these three functions in an overarching Program with maximum potential to benefit patients and the health care system overall.

BOX 1-2
Selected Milestones in U.S. Efforts to
Identify Effective Health Care Services

1930s   The U.S. Food and Drug Administration (FDA) is given authority to regulate the premarket review of new drugs for safety by the Federal Food, Drug, and Cosmetic Act (1938).

1960s   Technology assessment arises on the basis of the recognition that modern technology may have unintended, harmful consequences.

          The Kefauver-Harris Drug Amendments expand the FDA's responsibilities to include evaluations of safety and effectiveness. Effectiveness must be proved by "substantial evidence" (1962).

1970s   Congress gives the FDA significant authority through the Medical Device Amendments to regulate the testing and marketing of medical devices to ensure their safety and efficacy (1976).

          ECRI (now the ECRI Institute) publishes its first monthly publication dedicated to assessing medical technologies (1971).

          Congress establishes the U.S. Office of Technology Assessment (OTA) (P.L. 92-484) to perform objective analyses of technologies, including health care services, to aid policy making (1972). (Congress eliminated funding for OTA in 1995.)

          Wennberg and colleagues document wide variations in physician practices, making evident that the style of U.S. health care practice is likewise variable (1973).

          Congress establishes the National Center for Health Care Technology (P.L. 95-623) in 1978 to conduct medical technology assessments related to Medicare coverage decisions. (The program was dissolved in 1981 after Congress cut its funding.)

1980s   RAND Corporation researchers document that large proportions of the procedures that physicians perform are inappropriate, as judged by evidence-based decision criteria.

          The American College of Physicians initiates the Clinical Efficacy Assessment Project and begins publishing clinical guidelines (1981).

          The Veterans Administration institutes a Technology Assessment Committee to make recommendations on priority technologies for assessment and appropriate methods for technology assessment (1984).

          The Blue Cross and Blue Shield Association (BCBSA) establishes the Technology Evaluation Center to assess medical technologies through comprehensive reviews of clinical evidence (1985).

The Agency for Health Care Policy and Research (AHCPR) (now the Agency for Healthcare Research and Quality [AHRQ]) is created and given the responsibility for federal health services research by the Omnibus Budget Reconciliation Act of 1989 (P.L. 101-239). The agency's Center for Medical Effectiveness Research forms several Patient Outcome Research Teams to study the outcomes and costs of alternative treatments for specific clinical problems.

The Council of Medical Specialty Societies convenes a national meeting to promote guidelines and training programs for specialty societies and commissions the creation of a manual of evidence-based methods (1987).

Significant methodological advances enable the generation and use of evidence in medical decisions. These include decision trees, utility theory, Bayes theorem for analyzing diagnostic tests, mathematical models, cost-effectiveness analysis, clinical epidemiology, outcomes assessment, meta-analysis, and systematic review.

The U.S. Preventive Services Task Force (USPSTF) is convened in 1984 to evaluate research and issue guidelines for preventive interventions. It pioneers the use of comprehensive literature reviews and publishes the first *Guide to Clinical Preventive Services* in 1989.

1990s   AHCPR (now AHRQ) launches a program to create evidence-based guidelines (1990-1996).

The Cochrane Collaboration creates a network of organizations from 13 countries, including the United States, to promote evidence-based health care though the production of systematic reviews and clinical guidelines (1993).

Funding for AHCPR operations is seriously threatened in response to lobbying by a small group of orthopedic surgeons angered by a Patient Outcomes Research Team report on the treatment of back pain (1995-1996).

Congress eliminates funding for the Office of Technology Assessment (1995).

AHRQ establishes the Evidence-based Practice Centers (EPCs) program to produce reports on clinical evidence and technology assessments (1997).

AHRQ, the American Medical Association, and the American Association of Health Plans (now America's Health Insurance Plans) create the National Guideline Clearinghouse (1998).

Health plans, specialty societies, disease-based associations, and foundations create numerous programs that produce clinical guidelines.

The Centers for Medicare & Medicaid Services (CMS) establishes the Medicare Coverage Advisory Committee (now the Medicare Evidence Development and Coverage Advisory Committee) to provide objective assessments of the available evidence on the safety, efficacy, and clinical benefits of medical services or products for national coverage decisions (1998).

continued

BOX 1-2
Continued

2000s   CMS introduces Coverage with Evidence Development to generate data on the utilization and impacts of services being considered for a national Medicare coverage decision. The overall objective is to improve the evidence base for providers' recommendations to Medicare beneficiaries (2005).

AHRQ creates the Effective Health Care Program, authorized by Section 1013 of the Medicare Prescription Drug, Improvement, and Modernization Act of 2003 (P.L. 108-173) (2005).

The Institute of Medicine establishes the Roundtable on Evidence-Based Medicine (2006).

BCBSA, America's Health Insurance Plans, the Medicare Payment Advisory Commission, and others propose substantial new investment in comparative effectiveness research.

NOTE: The USPSTF was modeled on the Canadian Task Force on the Periodic Health Examination, which the Canadian Government created in 1976 to weigh the scientific evidence for and against using specific preventive services in asymptomatic populations (Canadian Task Force on Preventive Health Care, 2003).
SOURCES: Atkins et al. (2005); BCBSA (2007b); Canadian Task Force on Preventive Health Care (2003); CMS (2006); Congressional Research Service (2005); Eddy (2005); Gazelle et al. (2005); Gray et al. (2003); Helfand (2005); IOM (1985, 2006); Levin (2001); Steinberg and Luce (2005); USPSTF (2007).

Chapter 2, An Imperative for Change, documents the imperative for immediate action to change how the nation marshals clinical evidence and applies it to endorse the use of the most effective clinical interventions.

Chapter 3, Setting Priorities for Evidence Assessment, provides the committee's findings and recommendations on setting priorities for evidence assessment (systematic review) and describes key programmatic challenges in establishing a priority setting process for the Program.

Chapter 4, Systematic Reviews: The Central Link Between Evidence and Clinical Decision Making, reviews how high-quality evidence assessment (systematic review) is integral to identifying effective clinical services and presents the committee's recommendations for ensuring high-quality evidence assessment. Key programmatic challenges are highlighted.

Chapter 5, Developing Trusted Clinical Practice Guidelines, presents the committee's findings and recommendations for developing (or endorsing) standards for trusted clinical practice guidelines. Key programmatic challenges are highlighted.

Chapter 6, Building a Foundation for Knowing What Works in Health Care, considers how the previous chapters' recommendations may be best implemented. It provides guiding principles, assesses three basic alternatives, and recommends a general organizational framework for the Program. Key programmatic challenges are highlighted.

REFERENCES

America's Health Insurance Plans. 2007. *Setting a higher bar: We believe there is more the nation can do to improve quality and safety in health care.* Washington, DC: America's Health Insurance Plans.

Atkins, D., K. Fink, and J. Slutsky. 2005. Better information for better health care: The Evidence-based Practice Center program and the Agency for Healthcare Research and Quality. *Annals of Internal Medicine* 142(12 Part 2):1035-1041.

BCBSA (Blue Cross and Blue Shield Association). 2007a. *Blue Cross and Blue Shield Association proposes payer-funded institute to evaluate what medical treatments work best* http://www.bcbs.com/news/bcbsa/blue-cross-and-blue-shield-association-proposes-payer-funded-institute.html (accessed May 2007).

———. 2007b. *What is the Technology Evaluation Center?* http://www.bcbs.com/betterknowledge/tec/what-is-tec.html (accessed August 8, 2007).

Berwick, D. M. 2003. *Escape fire: Designs for the future of health care.* San Francisco, CA: Jossey-Bass.

Canadian Task Force on Preventive Health Care. 2003. *CTFPHC history/methodology* http://www.ctfphc.org (accessed July 24, 2007).

CMS (Centers for Medicare & Medicaid Services). 2006. *National coverage determinations with data collection as a condition of coverage: Coverage with evidence development* http://www.cms.hhs.gov/mcd/ncpc_view_document.asp?id=8 (accessed July 24, 2007).

Cochrane Collaboration. 2005. *Glossary of terms in the Cochrane Collaboration. Version 4.2.5* http://www.cochrane.org (accessed November 27, 2006).

Congressional Budget Office. 2007. Research on the comparative effectiveness of medical treatments: Options for an expanded federal role. *Testimony by Director Peter R. Orszag before House Ways and Means Subcommittee on Health* http://www.cbo.gov/ftpdocs/82xx/doc8209/Comparative_Testimony.pdf (accessed June 12, 2007).

Congressional Research Service. 2005. *Technology assessment in Congress: History and legislative options, CRS report to Congress.* Washington, DC: Library of Congress.

Dictionary.com. 2007. Results for "evidence." *Dictionary.com Unabridged (v 1.1)* http://dictionary.reference.com/browse/evidence (accessed October 2, 2007).

Eddy, D. M. 2005. Evidence-based medicine: A unified approach. *Health Affairs* 24(1):9-17.

Fisher, E. S., and J. E. Wennberg. 2003. Health care quality, geographic variations, and the challenge of supply-sensitive care. *Perspectives in Biology and Medicine* 46(1):69-79.

Fisher, E. S., D. E. Wennberg, T. A. Stukel, D. J. Gottlieb, F. L. Lucas, and E. L. Pinder. 2003a. The implications of regional variations in Medicare spending. Part 1: The content, quality, and accessibility of care. *Annals of Internal Medicine* 138(4):273.

———. 2003b. The implications of regional variations in Medicare spending. Part 2: Health outcomes and satisfaction with care. *Annals of Internal Medicine* 138(4):288.

Gabel, J. R., A. T. Lo Sasso, and T. Rice. 2002. Consumer-driven health plans: Are they more than talk now? *Health Affairs* w2.395.

Gazelle, G. S., P. M. McMahon, U. Siebert, and M. T. Beinfeld. 2005. Cost-effectiveness analysis in the assessment of diagnostic imaging technologies. *Radiology* 235(2):361-370.

Glasziou, P., and B. Haynes. 2005. The paths from research to improved health outcomes. *ACP Journal Club* 142(2):A8-A10.

Gray, B. H. 1992. The legislative battle over health services research. *Health Affairs* 11(4): 38-66.

Gray, B. H., M. K. Gusmano, and S. Collins. 2003. AHCPR and the changing politics of health services research. *Health Affairs* w3.283.

Haynes, R. B., D. L. Sackett, G. H. Guyatt, and P. Tugwell. 2006. *Clinical epidemiology: How to do clinical practice research.* 3rd ed. Philadelphia, PA: Lipincott Williams & Wilkins.

The Health Industry Forum. 2006. *Comparative effectiveness forum: Key themes.* Washington, DC: The Health Industry Forum.

Helfand, M. 2005. Using evidence reports: Progress and challenges in evidence-based decision making. *Health Affairs* 24(1):123-127.

Higgins, J. T., and S. Green. 2006. *Cochrane handbook for systematic reviews of interventions 4.2.6 [updated September 2006],* The Cochrane Library, Issue 4, 2006. Chichester, UK: John Wiley & Sons, Ltd.

IOM (Institute of Medicine). 1985. *Assessing medical technologies.* Washington, DC: National Academy Press.

———. 2001. *Crossing the quality chasm: A new health system for the 21st century.* Washington, DC: National Academy Press.

———. 2006. *Safe medical devices for children.* Edited by Field, M. J., and H. Tilson. Washington, DC: The National Academies Press.

———. 2007. *Learning what works best: The nation's need for evidence on comparative effectiveness in health care* http://www.iom.edu/ebm-effectiveness (accessed April 2007).

Khan, K. S., G. ter Riet, J. Popay, J. Nixon, and J. Kleijnen. 2001. Stage II conducting the review: Phase 5 study quality assessment. In *CRD Report Number 4.* Edited by Khan, K. S., G. ter Riet, H. Glanville, A. J. Sowden, and J. Kleijnen. York, UK: NHS Centre for Reviews and Dissemination, University of York.

Last, J. M. 2001. *A dictionary of epidemiology.* New York: Oxford University Press.

Levin, A. 2001. The Cochrane Collaboration. *Annals of Internal Medicine* 135(4):309-312.

Lomas, J., T. Culyer, C. McCutcheon, L. McAuley, and L. Law. 2005. *Conceptualizing and combining evidence for health system guidance.* Ottawa (Ontario): Canadian Health Services Research Foundation.

Lumpkin, J. R. 2006. *Presentation to the HECS Committee Meeting, July 24, 2006.* Washington, DC.

McGlynn, E. A., S. M. Asch, J. Adams, J. Keesey, J. Hicks, A. DeCristofaro, and E. A. Kerr. 2003. The quality of health care delivered to adults in the United States. *The New England Journal of Medicine* 348(26):2635-2645.

Medicare Payment Advisory Commission. 2005. Chapter 8: Using clinical and cost effectiveness in Medicare. In *Report to the Congress: Issues in a modernized Medicare* http://www.medpac.gov/documents/June05_Entire_report.pdf (accessed June 2007).

———. 2007. Chapter 2: Producing comparative effectiveness information. In *Report to the Congress: Promoting greater efficiency in Medicare* http://www.medpac.gov/documents/Jun07_EntireReport.pdf (accessed June 2007).

Mulrow, C., and K. Lohr. 2001. Proof and policy from medical research evidence. *Journal of Health Politics, Policy and Law* 26(2):249-266.

Rettig, R., P. Jacobsen, C. Farquhar, and W. Aubrey. 2007. *False hope: Bone marrow transplantation for breast cancer.* New York: Oxford University Press.

Sackett, D. L., W. M. C. Rosenberg, J. A. M. Gray, R. B. Haynes, and W. S. Richardson. 1996. Evidence based medicine: What it is and what it isn't. *BMJ* 312(7023):71-72.

Schwartz, J. S. 1984. The role of professional medical societies in reducing practice variations. *Health Affairs* 3(2):90-101.

Steinberg, E. P., and B. R. Luce. 2005. Evidence based? Caveat emptor! *Health Affairs* 24(1):80-92.

Straus, S. E., P. Glasziou, W. S. Richardson, and R. B. Haynes. 2005. *Evidence-based medicine: How to practice and teach EBM.* 3rd ed. London, UK: Churchill Livingstone.

U.S. Government Accountability Office. 2006a. *Consumer-directed health plans: Small but growing enrollment fueled by rising cost of health care coverage.* GAO-06-514. Washington, DC: Government Printing Office.

———. 2006b. *Employee compensation: Employer spending on benefits has grown faster than wages, due largely to rising costs for health insurance and retirement benefits.* GAO-06-285. Washington, DC: Government Printing Office.

USPSTF (U.S. Preventive Services Task Force). 2007. *About USPSTF* http://www.ahrq.gov/clinic/uspstfab.htm (accessed July 28, 2007).

Webster, P. 2006. US big businesses struggle to cope with health-care costs. *Lancet* 367(9505): 101-102.

Wennberg, J. E. 2002. Unwarranted variations in healthcare delivery: Implications for academic medical centres. *BMJ* 325(7370):961-964.

———. 2004. Perspective: Practice variations and health care reform: Connecting the dots. *Health Affairs* var.140.

West, S., V. King, T. Carey, K. Lohr, N. McCoy, S. Sutton, and L. Lux. 2002. *Systems to rate the strength of scientific evidence. Evidence Report/Technology Assessment No. 47.* (Prepared by the Research Triangle Institute-University of North Carolina Evidence-based Practice Center under Contract No. 290-97-0011.) AHRQ Publication No. 02-E016. Rockville, MD: Agency for Healthcare Research and Quality.

Wilensky, G. R. 2006. Developing a center for comparative effectiveness information. *Health Affairs* w572.

2

An Imperative for Change

Abstract: This chapter documents the imperative for immediate action to change how the nation marshals clinical evidence and applies it to endorse the most effective clinical interventions. The chapter describes five interconnecting, persistent health policy challenges that are inextricably associated with the need to know what works in health care: (1) unsustainable rates of increase in costs, (2) unwarranted geographic variation in the use of services, (3) unreliable quality, (4) consumer-directed health care, and (5) the need to make informed decisions about the health services that should be covered by health insurance. The chapter provides a brief description and assessment of the efforts that are being made to address the need for information on clinical effectiveness as well as the primary challenges facing the current system. This sets the stage for the committee's recommendations for addressing the challenge in the subsequent chapters.

To a great extent, the resolution of some of the nation's most pressing health policy concerns hinges on the capacity to identify highly effective clinical services. Unsustainable rates of growth in health spending result from the delivery of effective as well as ineffective care. The high costs associated with the provision of both appropriate and inappropriate care lead to higher insurance premiums. Unwarranted variation in clinical practice reflects deviations from accepted standards of care, as well as uncertainty and disagreement regarding what those standards should be. This contributes to the health care quality chasm in which patients cannot always be assured that they will receive the best, most effective care. The common thread in each of these policy areas is the need to differentiate between effective and ineffective care.

In recent years, the capacity of the United States to evaluate clinical effectiveness has improved substantially. A number of public and private organizations synthesize and assess the evidence on clinical effectiveness, and many others focus on applying in real world settings the knowledge that those organizations generate. However, significant gaps in the ability to develop, synthesize, and apply the evidence on clinical effectiveness remain; and the nation faces major challenges as an array of new—and often very expensive—technologies and treatments rapidly enter the health care marketplace. As a result, the nation needs to continue to improve its capacity to assess clinical effectiveness and ensure that health care decision making is grounded in the evidence about what works.

BACKGROUND

Over the past 50 years medical knowledge has grown dramatically as breakthroughs have occurred in numerous areas of medical science, including genomics, stem cell biology, biomedical engineering, molecular biology, and immunology (Sung et al., 2003). Investments in biomedical research, both public and private, have increased steadily over time, resulting in a rapid pace of innovation in health care (Neumann and Sandberg, 1998; Zinner, 2001). Many more preventive, diagnostic, and treatment alternatives are available to patients than were available in past years; and even more are in development, including products that have resulted from research in pharmacogenomics, biotechnology, and nanotechnology (Joint Economic Committee, 2007; Walsh, 2005). Investments in research directed at understanding the human genome and the functions of genes will provide more opportunities to deliver personalized medicine, which will tailor diagnoses and therapies to an individual's own genotype (Meadows, 2005).

At the same time, the 77 million members of the nation's baby boom generation are nearing retirement age, and soon the health system will be confronted with patients from this large and increasingly complex cohort of individuals with multiple comorbidities, including physical and cognitive impairments (AHRQ, 2001). This will place increased demands on the health system and will add to cost pressures.

For patients and providers, as well as for society as a whole, ascertaining the effectiveness of the available preventive, diagnostic, and treatment options is becoming increasingly urgent. The expense of emerging technologies and the projected increases in consumer demand virtually ensure that cost control will be a central focus for policy makers, health plans, and others in the coming years (Clancy, 2003). Moreover, variation in treatment patterns means that, in many cases, patients will continue to receive care that deviates from standards of high quality. In the context of rapidly rising costs, society's ability to distinguish between health interventions that work and those that do not work, and for whom they work, is becoming more and more important.

Medical Advances

In recent years, many new diagnostics, devices, drugs, biologics, and procedures have been added to the medical armamentarium. In addition, innovations first established in other fields have been applied to medicine through technology transfer, including lasers, ultrasound, and magnetic resonance spectroscopy (Gelijns and Rosenberg, 1994).

Over the course of the coming decade, the pace of innovation in medical care is likely to accelerate even more. Although the time from discovery to clinical availability remains long, many medical innovations are moving closer to the release stage. In recent years, the number of patents that have been issued for biomedical devices and biopharmaceuticals has increased significantly. From 1991 to 2003, the number of new patents issued for medical devices doubled from 4,500 to more than 9,000. From 1992 to 2001, the total number of biotechnology patents granted per year tripled, from less than 2,600 to nearly 7,800 (IOM, 2007a).

Information Overload

Along with the increase in the numbers of medical treatments and interventions that are available, the volume of literature describing investigations of these interventions has also expanded. From 1978 to 2001, 8.1 million journal articles were published in MEDLINE.[1] From 1978 to 1985, the average annual number of articles indexed by MEDLINE was 272,344. By the 1994 to 2001 time period, the average annual volume of indexed articles had increased by 46 percent to 442,756. Much of the growth in the literature was in articles on randomized trials and other types of clinical research that could be used to guide evidence-based practice (Druss and Marcus, 2005).

The evidence base for clinical effectiveness has thus become so vast that it is essentially unmanageable for individual providers (IOM, 2001). Yet, at the same time, the primary literature provides limited guidance on a broad range of urgent clinical questions, such as comparative effectiveness and long-term patient outcomes (Tunis et al., 2003).

The massive quantity of evidence places significant demands on anyone

---

[1] MEDLINE is a database of the National Library of Medicine, National Institutes of Health.

seeking to stay abreast of current standards of care. For physicians, information on the available care options can be overwhelming, even when just a single class of interventions, such as pharmaceuticals, is considered. For example, for antihypertensive medications, a search of the PubMed database of the National Center for Biotechnology Information of the National Library of Medicine, the National Institutes of Health (NIH) (http://pubmed. gov), by use of the terms "antihypertensive agents AND therapeutic use" identified 312 English-language review articles that the PubMed database had indexed between October 1, 2006, and September 12, 2007.

As a result of this increase in the quantity of relevant information, synthesized information such as systematic reviews, clinical guidelines, and resources (e.g., *The Cochrane Library*), have become essential tools for the users of the evidence (Druss and Marcus, 2005). However, the number of these products has also grown substantially. For example, as of September 2007, the Agency for Healthcare Research and Quality's (AHRQ's) National Guideline Clearinghouse (2007b) listed 54 clinical practice guidelines under the heading "antihypertensives." In this situation, end users need a mechanism to determine which summaries are the most relevant, valid, and reliable.

For physicians—and patients—who are motivated enough to read through and assess all of the relevant individual clinical studies on their own, keeping current is an arduous, if not impossible, task. Given the variable quality of the research and its limited generalizability, these providers and patients are faced not only with reconciling vastly different research findings but also with scrutinizing each study's methodology in detail to ensure that the study has been well designed, that the analyses have been well performed, and that the results apply to their particular clinical circumstance (Abramson, 2004). This expectation is unrealistic, especially given that today's medical residents frequently lack the knowledge in biostatistics necessary to interpret the findings of published clinical research (Windish et al., 2007). These findings illustrate the need for a system that can make sense of all of the data that currently exist, as well as the new knowledge that is now being generated.

PERSISTENT HEALTH POLICY CHALLENGES

Clinical effectiveness is a central issue in health care. Improving the capacity to conduct clinical effectiveness assessments has the potential to improve health care in a range of vital areas, from cost to quality and access. These opportunities make it imperative that the United States makes improvements in its capacity to make impartial, accurate effectiveness assessments. This capability may also provide the financial leeway needed to allow the adoption of innovative breakthrough technologies.

Unsustainable Rates of Increase in Costs

A significant proportion of health care costs is directed to care that has not been shown to be effective and that may actually be harmful. For example, Wennberg and colleagues (2006) concluded that decreased utilization of acute care hospitals and physician visits by Medicare beneficiaries could actually lead to better clinical outcomes and also prolong the solvency of the program. The authors found that 30 percent of Medicare spending on chronically ill individuals was unnecessary. Other studies have also estimated that the potential savings from reducing excessive spending on services of little or no value in the Medicare program may be as high as 30 percent of all expenditures (Wennberg et al., 2002a).

Historically, health care cost-containment efforts in the United States have had little to no success (Altman and Levitt, 2002). The levels of spending on health care rose from 5.7 percent of the gross domestic product (GDP) in 1965 to 16 percent of the GDP in 2004 (Lubitz, 2005). By 2015, spending is projected to reach 20 percent of the GDP, or an estimated $4 trillion, up from $1.9 trillion in 2004 (Borger et al., 2006; Cutler, 2005). The U.S. Government Accountability Office (2007) concludes that rising health care costs pose a fiscal challenge not just to the federal budget but also to states, American businesses, and society as a whole.

The federal Medicare program spent $374 billion in 2006 and accounted for 13 percent of all federal spending (Kaiser Family Foundation, 2007). Spending on Medicare is projected to reach $564 billion in 2012 and in the subsequent years will continue to consume an increasingly large portion of federal revenues. Along with projected increases in spending on Social Security, Medicaid, and interest on the federal debt, these expenditures will begin to crowd out spending in many other areas of the budget. As a result, fiscal pressures will necessitate a series of difficult budget decisions in coming years (Walker, 2007). Figure 2-1 provides Congressional Budget Office estimates of Medicare and Medicaid spending as a percentage of the GDP through 2050. In this context, improving the U.S. capacity to evaluate the effectiveness of medical treatment options appears to be vital.

Unwarranted Geographic Variation in the Use of Health Services

Evidence suggests that there is a substantial potential to improve the quality of health care by addressing the inappropriate variation in the use of health services (IOM, 2001). Analysis of the widespread geographic differences in health spending and the use of services does not support the hypothesis that greater spending results in increased life expectancy or better health outcomes overall in the regions with higher levels of spending (Fisher et al., 2003a; Fuchs, 2004; Wennberg et al., 2002b).

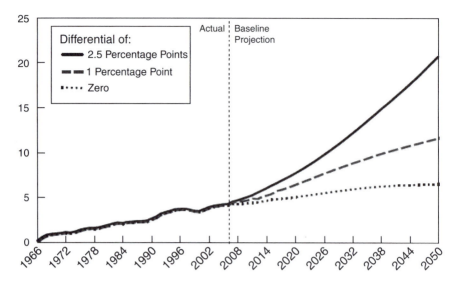

FIGURE 2-1 Total federal spending for Medicare and Medicaid under assumptions about the health care cost growth differential.
SOURCE: Congressional Budget Office (2007).

Health care differs substantially across the country, from one small region to another and from one city to the next (Feenberg and Skinner, 2000; Fisher et al., 2003a). These variations occur across a wide range of health interventions, including the use of delivery by cesarean section (Baicker et al., 2006); cardiac procedures after acute myocardial infarction (Guadagnoli et al., 1995); treatment of degenerative diseases of the hip, knee, and spine (Weinstein et al., 2004); and the treatment of individuals who are chronically ill (Wennberg et al., 2004). There are also significant disparities in the quality and the quantity of the health services received by minority groups in the United States (IOM, 2003).

Among Medicare beneficiaries, regional differences in spending reflect a greater frequency of physician visits, the more frequent use of specialist consultations, more frequent tests and minor procedures, and the greater use of the hospital and intensive care unit in certain regions (Fisher et al., 2003b). In addition, larger expenditures are associated with dramatic differences in end-of-life care seen in various parts of the country (Skinner and Wennberg, 2003). Overall, the difference in lifetime Medicare spending between a typical 65-year-old in Miami, Florida, and one in Minneapolis, Minnesota, has been estimated to be more than $50,000 (Wennberg et al., 2002b). Figure 2-2 illustrates these spending differentials in 2003.

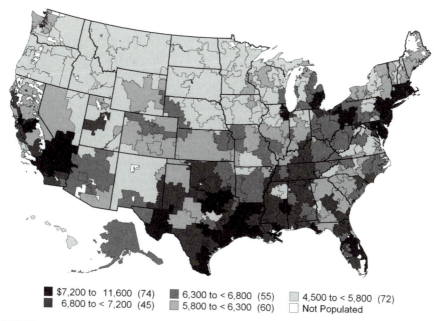

FIGURE 2-2 Medicare spending per capita in the United States, by hospital referral region, 2003.
NOTE: The numbers in parentheses indicate the number of regions in each group. Reprinted, with permission, from *The Dartmouth Atlas Project*, 2003. Copyright 2007 by The Trustees of Dartmouth College.
SOURCE: The Dartmouth Atlas Project (2003).

Greater expenditures do not necessarily result in better health outcomes, however (Fuchs, 2004). Fisher and colleagues (2003b) found no evidence that the patterns of practice observed in higher-spending regions led to improved survival, a slower decline in functional status, or a greater satisfaction with care. A higher rate of utilization of medical tests and procedures can, in some cases, have negative consequences for patients, as in the case of false-positive screening test results (Mitka, 2004). Consequently, differentiating between effective and ineffective health utilization is an important policy objective.

Variation in physician practice patterns has been a persistent concern because it points to the overuse and underuse of specific health services (Schwartz, 1984; Wennberg, 2004). These designations suggest that there are benchmarks that define optimal use; however, these are often not well defined. Investigators have asserted that, for some preference sensitive services, informed patient preference should be used to establish the benchmarks for appropriate use (Wennberg, 1988; Wennberg and Wennberg, 2003), yet this presupposes that patients (and providers) have access to reliable, relevant, and trustworthy information about treatment outcomes. This is often not the case. As a result, many policy makers have called for the establishment of a national organization that would be able to meet the need for clinical effectiveness information (America's Health Insurance Plans, 2007; BCBSA, 2007a; Medicare Payment Advisory Commission, 2007; Shortell et al., 2007; Wilensky, 2006).

The Quality Chasm

The Institute of Medicine (IOM) report *Crossing the Quality Chasm* (2001) identified six aims for patient care: safety, effectiveness, patient centeredness, timeliness, efficiency, and equity. To promote effective care, the report indicated that scientific knowledge should be employed to ensure that all patients who might benefit from a certain intervention receive the services, whereas those who are not likely to benefit should not (i.e., avoiding underuse and overuse). The report recognized that the evidence base needed to support effective care is limited for many health and health care topics, but it concluded that health care providers and organizations should do more to determine the most appropriate therapies on the basis of the strength of the evidence and then adhere to those preferred therapies.

Strategies that encourage quality improvement, such as pay-for-performance incentives, are also based on the ability to recognize excellent performance, promote best practices, and reduce errors (Berwick et al., 2003). The IOM report *Rewarding Provider Performance* (2007b) highlights performance measures as key building blocks in this effort. However, these measures must be based on benchmarks of appropriate clinical performance, and these are often not available. Thus, a lack of reliable information about clinical effectiveness limits the ability to guide care and to evaluate it.

Consumer-Directed Health Care

Many policy makers believe in empowering consumers and patients to be prudent managers of their own health and health care (Buntin et al., 2006; Congressional Budget Office, 2006). Proponents of consumer-directed health plans argue that consumers who are equipped with good information on the cost and quality of health services will have the power to reduce the cost and improve the quality of care. Yet, information on the effectiveness, risks, and benefits of alternative treatments is rarely adequate (U.S. Government Accountability Office, 2006).

Coverage Decisions

Private and public health plans are struggling with an almost daily challenge of learning how their covered populations might benefit—or be harmed—by newly available health services. In making coverage decisions, it is rare for plans to have access to all of the information that they need, and it is often unclear what should guide their decision making in cases in which the scientific knowledge is inconclusive or lacking. Determining what level of evidence and what degree of certainty is sufficient to move forward with a decision to cover or not cover a new treatment involves a judgment about the risks of acting too soon (promoting the use of a treatment that is later determined to be ineffective or harmful) and acting too late (delaying the use of a treatment that is truly beneficial) (Atkins et al., 2005b).

The value of costly, emerging technologies is widely debated. Cutler and McClellan (2001) argue that although technological changes have accounted for the bulk of the increases in medical expenditures over time, these medical advances have proved to be worth far more than their costs. In contrast, Redberg (2007) argues that many treatments undergo rapid adoption despite relatively limited evidence, resulting in high levels of spending for unproven procedures. The current controversy over the use of drug-eluting stents for the treatment of vascular disease is a case in point.

In deciding what to include as part of their covered package of benefits, health plans and purchasers must decide about the value of specific interventions for particular groups of patients. Health services and technologies are deemed medically necessary, and therefore appropriate for inclusion in the benefit package, or experimental and investigational, and therefore not eligible for coverage. However, the term "medical necessity" is ill defined, unexamined, and idiosyncratically applied (Berghold, 1995). Historically, insurers relied on the expert opinions of physicians in deciding what services and technologies to include as part of their benefit packages. Over time, however, plans have placed a stronger emphasis on high-quality scientific studies (Garber, 2001; Tunis and Pearson, 2006).

CURRENT LANDSCAPE

Providers, patients, health plans, and others need information about clinical effectiveness to ensure that the decisions that they make are solidly grounded in the evidence about what works. Toward that end, Congress has substantially increased funding for the NIH in recent years. Between 1998 and 2003 the NIH budget doubled, and by fiscal year 2007 it had reached $28.6 billion (Loscalzo, 2006). Private spending on research has also increased significantly (Iglehart, 2001). For example, investments in research and development on new medicines by the biotechnology and pharmaceutical research member companies of the Pharmaceutical Research and Manufacturers of America (PhRMA) (2006) reached $39.4 billion in 2005, up from $2 billion in 1980.

In recent years there have also been increasing investments in the synthesis of the available clinical evidence in the United States, for example, with the establishment of AHRQ's Evidence-based Practice Centers (EPCs), as well as private-sector activities (Atkins et al., 2005a; Garber, 2001). Appropriations for health services research made to all federal agencies— AHRQ, the NIH, the Veteran's Health Administration, the U.S. Department of Defense, the Centers for Medicare & Medicaid Services (CMS), the U.S. Food and Drug Administration (FDA), and the Centers for Disease Control and Prevention—has now reached approximately $1.5 billion annually. However, research on clinical effectiveness receives only a small part of that investment (IOM, 2007a). In general, vastly more funding is available for primary medical research than for the synthesis of the available evidence.

Key Players

A number of public- and private-sector organizations are involved in the collection, analysis, and dissemination of clinical effectiveness information. In addition to the NIH and the private-sector groups that fund primary research, many other organizations are involved in assessing that information and synthesizing it in ways that inform decision making. Some of the many organizations that conduct these activities are described below.

U.S. Food and Drug Administration

In deciding whether particular drugs or devices should be allowed to enter the market, the FDA plays a central role in assessing clinical efficacy data. The FDA consists of eight offices. One of these, the Center for Drug Evaluation and Research (CDER), evaluates the safety and efficacy of all new drugs before they are sold on the market and monitors the safety of drugs after they have been approved. Other offices within the FDA include the Center for Biologics Evaluation and Research and the Center for Devices and Radiological Health.

In deciding on drug approvals, the CDER relies on advisory committees to obtain outside opinions and advice. Advisory committees review the evidence and provide input on new drugs; major new indications for previously approved drugs; and requirements for new drugs, such as boxed warnings on drug labels. The CDER takes advisory committee recommendations under consideration, but they are not binding (CDER, 2007). The CDER follows many of the same procedures when it evaluates its portfolio of new products, which include vaccines and blood- and tissue-derived products.

The process for obtaining FDA approval for devices is entirely different from the process for obtaining approval for drugs, and the standards for proving safety and efficacy are also different. All medical devices must be manufactured under a quality assurance program, be suitable for the intended use, be adequately packaged and properly labeled, and have establishment registration and device listing forms on file with the FDA. The manufacturers of only some classes of devices, however, must provide clinical data showing safety and efficacy.

AHRQ's Effective Health Care Program

Under Section 1013 of the Medicare Prescription Drug, Improvement, and Modernization Act, Congress directed AHRQ to conduct and support research focused on patient outcomes; comparative clinical effectiveness; and the appropriateness of specific pharmaceuticals, devices, and health services. This AHRQ project, known as the Effective Health Care Program, incorporates three approaches as part of its work on comparative effectiveness: (1) knowledge synthesis through the EPCs (see below); (2) the generation of new knowledge through a network of research-based health care organizations with access to electronic health information databases and the capacity to conduct rapid-turnaround research; and (3) the translation of the research work into patient-oriented materials, conducted through the John M. Eisenberg Clinical Decisions and Communications Science Center (AHRQ, 2007b). Congress has appropriated $15 million annually for this effort.

Syntheses of the Available Evidence

Public and private organizations, such as AHRQ's EPCs, the Blue Cross and Blue Shield Association (BCBSA) Technology Evaluation Center (TEC), the Cochrane Collaboration, the ECRI Institute, and Hayes, Inc., conduct syntheses of the available evidence (Table 2-1). These organizations provide systematic reviews, meta-analyses, and technology assessments that synthesize the available literature and describe what is known about the effectiveness of specific clinical interventions.

Individuals and organizations use the syntheses of the available evidence that these organizations produce in a number of ways. Public and private health plans use the information to inform their coverage decisions, professional and patient care organizations use the information to create practice guidelines, organizations that track provider performance rely on it to establish benchmarks of appropriate care, and the information is also

TABLE 2-1 Examples of Organizations That Conduct Evidence Syntheses

Organization	Description
AHRQ EPCs	In 1997, AHRQ launched an initiative establishing 12 EPCs in an effort to promote evidence-based practice in everyday care. AHRQ awards five-year contracts to EPCs to develop evidence reports and technology assessments. Currently, there are 13 EPCs in both university and private settings.
BCBSA TEC	BCBSA founded TEC in 1985 to provide decision makers with objective assessments of clinical effectiveness. TEC serves a wide range of clients in both the private and the public sectors, including Kaiser Permanente and CMS. Assessments are reviewed by the Medical Advisory Panel, consisting of experts in various specialties. TEC is a designated EPC, and its products are publicly available on its website.
Cochrane Collaboration	The Cochrane Collaboration is an independent, nonprofit organization that produces and disseminates systematic reviews of health care interventions. Founded in 1993, Cochrane is the largest and best known multinational organization working to evaluate health interventions based on systematic reviews. Its reviews are prepared by health professionals and others, including consumers, who work as part of one or more of the 51 Cochrane Review Groups. Editorial teams oversee the preparation and maintenance of the reviews and the application of quality standards, as documented in a regularly updated *Handbook*. Cochrane's contributors are funded from a variety of sources including governments, home institutions, and private funds. Commercial funding of review groups, centers, and the annual Colloquium is not allowed, however. Cochrane is also funded through royalties emanating from subscriptions to *The Cochrane Library*. Cochrane review abstracts, and plain language summaries are made available to the public for free and complete reviews are available via subscription to *The Cochrane Library*, which includes a variety of databases of reviews and controlled trials. The *Cochrane Database of Systematic Reviews*, the most important of these, included more than 4,900 protocols and reviews as of Issue 3, 2007.
ECRI Institute	The ECRI Institute is a nonprofit organization that provides technology assessments and cost-effectiveness analyses to ECRI Institute members and clients, including hospitals; health systems; public and private payers; U.S. federal and state government agencies; and ministries of health, voluntary sector organizations, associations, and accrediting agencies. Its products and methods are generally not available to the public. The ECRI Institute is a designated EPC and is also a Collaborating Center of the World Health Organization.
Hayes, Inc.	Hayes, Inc., is a for-profit organization, established in 1989, to develop health technology assessments for health organizations, including health plans, managed care companies, hospitals, and health networks. Hayes, Inc., produces several professional products, including the *Hayes Briefs*, the *Hayes Directory*, and the *Hayes Outlook*. Its products and methods are generally not available to the public.

SOURCES: AHRQ (2007c); BCBSA (2007b); Cochrane Collaboration (2007); ECRI Institute (2007); Hayes, Inc. (2007).

employed by other researchers and the general public. Table 2-2 describes several of the ways in which public-sector organizations use the evidence synthesis.

Clinical Guideline Developers

Another way in which evidence syntheses may be applied in practice is through the development of clinical guidelines and recommendations. Medical professional societies, patient advocacy groups, trade associations, and others have instituted processes to collect and analyze evidence (including systematic reviews) and develop clinical recommendations on the basis of that information (Table 2-3). Almost 2,200 guidelines are now included in the National Guideline Clearinghouse, which is supported by AHRQ (NGC, 2007a).

Many consider the U.S. Preventive Services Task Force (USPSTF) to be a model for clinical recommendation development. The USPSTF conducts

TABLE 2-2 Public-Sector Activities That Use Evidence Syntheses

Organization	Description
CMS MedCAC	CMS established MCAC (now MedCAC) in 1998 to provide independent expert advice to CMS on specific clinical topics. MedCAC reviews and evaluates the medical literature and technology assessments on medical items and services that are under evaluation at CMS. MedCAC can be an integral part of the national coverage determination process. MedCAC is advisory in nature; CMS is responsible for all final decisions.
DERP	DERP is a collaboration of public and private organizations, including 13 state programs, that develops reports assessing the comparative effectiveness and safety of drugs within particular drug classes. EPCs conduct evidence reviews for DERP. State Medicaid programs have used this information to develop their drug formularies.
NIH CDP	The CDP conferences convene independent panels of researchers, health professionals, and public representatives who consider the literature reviews conducted by EPCs, as well as expert testimony. The NIH staff select clinical topics on the basis of their public health importance, their prevalence, controversy over the topics, the potential to reduce gaps between knowledge and practice, the availability of scientific information, and the impact of the individual topics on health care costs. The CDP produces consensus statements not intended to serve as practice guidelines.

NOTE: CDP = Consensus Development Program; DERP = Drug Effectiveness Review Project; MCAC = Medicare Coverage Advisory Committee; MedCAC = Medicare Evidence Development and Coverage Advisory Committee.
SOURCES: CMS (2006, 2007b); DERP (2007); NIH Consensus Development Program (2007).

TABLE 2-3 Examples of Organizations That Establish Clinical
Guidelines and Recommendations

Organization	Description
ACC/AHA	The ACC has partnered with the AHA to develop guidelines for evidence-based cardiovascular care since 1980. Writing groups are specifically charged with performing a formal literature review, weighing the strength of evidence for or against a particular treatment or procedure, and including estimates of expected health outcomes when data exist.
ACP	In 1981, the ACP launched the Clinical Efficacy Assessment Project to evaluate advances in medicine and develop clinical practice guidelines based on the best evidence available. Current guidelines are based on evidence reports commissioned by AHRQ and produced by EPCs.
ADA	The ADA has established the Evidence Analysis Library, which consists of relevant nutritional research and evidence-based guidelines.
AHRQ and USPSTF	The U.S. Public Health Service convened USPSTF in 1984, and since 1998 it has been sponsored by AHRQ. The USPSTF consists of a panel of private-sector experts, and its recommendations are regarded as the "gold standard" for clinical preventive services.
American Diabetes Association	The American Diabetes Association funds research, publishes scientific findings, and conducts programs nationwide. Clinical practice guidelines and recommendations are developed from literature reviews by clinicians and are reviewed by the Executive Committee.
ASCO	ASCO convenes expert panels to develop clinical practice guidelines for methods of cancer treatment and care. The manual for generating these guidelines is updated regularly to reflect significant changes.
NHLBI	The NHLBI organizes voluntary expert panels to develop clinical practice guidelines related to heart, blood vessel, lung, and blood diseases in children and adults.

NOTE: ACC = American College of Cardiology; ACP = American College of Physicians; ADA = American Dietetic Association; AHA = American Heart Association; ASCO = American Society of Clinical Oncology; NHLBI = National Heart, Lung, and Blood Institute.
SOURCES: ACC (2007); ACP (2007); ADA (2007); AHRQ (2007a); American Diabetes Association (2007); ASCO (2007); Eagle and Guyton (2004); NHLBI (2007).

impartial assessments of the scientific evidence to reach conclusions about the effectiveness of a broad range of clinical preventive services, including screening, counseling, and preventive medications. Its recommendations are intended for use in the primary care setting.

Under contract to AHRQ, an EPC conducts systematic reviews of the evidence on specific topics in clinical prevention that serve as the scientific basis for USPSTF recommendations. The USPSTF reviews the EPC report, estimates the magnitude of benefits and harms for each preventive service, reaches consensus about the net benefit for each preventive service, and issues a recommendation.

Performance Measurement Organizations

A number of organizations track and evaluate provider performance by measuring their actual clinical practices against the recommended practices (Table 2-4). To conduct this work, performance measurement groups first establish standards of care against which the performance of providers can be assessed. These are based on the available evidence and the guidelines issued by professional groups. In many cases, however, adequate guidelines are not available or are not evidence based, and this has been a significant barrier to the development of performance measures.

Significant Challenges

Although the U.S. system for the development, synthesis, and application of clinical evidence has expanded and improved over the past several decades, it continues to face significant challenges. Among these are the persistent gaps in the information available to decision makers, as well as the confusing manner in which the information is presented (e.g., different organizations use different coding schemes to represent similar concepts). Moreover, the quality of the information is often suspect because of a lack of transparency regarding the methods used to generate the information as well as conflict of interest concerns. In addition, inefficiencies in the current system that result from duplications of effort mean that fewer resources are available to fill the remaining information gaps. These concerns are detailed below.

Unmet Information Needs

Physicians now have access to a vast amount of relevant clinical information, but often this information is difficult to navigate and it may not address their specific concerns (Tunis, 2005). New tools, such as the Up-to-Date database and the American College of Physicians' Physicians' Information and Education Resource are bringing more information directly to physicians' offices, but uncertainties about the quality and the applicability of the evidence remain.

The available information may not be suitable to the clinician's needs for a number of reasons. For example, although the provider may want to

TABLE 2-4 Examples of Organizations That Measure Performance

Organization	Description
AQA Alliance	In 2004, the American Academy of Family Physicians, the American College of Physicians, and America's Health Insurance Plans joined with AHRQ to create the AQA Alliance (originally the Ambulatory Care Quality Alliance). The AQA Alliance has developed a collaborative process in which physicians, consumers, purchasers, health insurance plans, and others develop strategies for measuring performance at the physician or group level; collecting data; and reporting the information to consumers, physicians, and other stakeholders.
The Joint Commission (formerly JCAHO)	A nonprofit organization established in 1951, the Joint Commission evaluates 15,000 health organizations in the United States and provides accreditation to those meeting its quality standards. The Joint Commission sets standards to ensure the quality and the safety of the care provided. Performance measures supplement the standards-based survey process by providing specific performance targets, allowing ongoing performance monitoring, and working toward continuous improvement.
NCQA	A nonprofit organization founded in 1990, the NCQA accredits health organizations to provide consumers and employers with an indicator of quality. The NCQA develops quality standards and performance measures, building consensus among large employers, policy makers, physicians, patients, and health plans to decide what aspects of quality to measure, how to measure it, and how to promote improvement. The NCQA tracks quality through the Health Plan Employer Data and Information Set and publishes annual reports on its findings.
NQF	A nonprofit membership organization founded in 1999, the NQF was established as a public-private partnership to promote a common approach to measuring and reporting health care quality. The NQF includes participation from consumers, public and private purchasers, employers, professionals, provider organizations, health plans, accrediting bodies, and others. Its goals are to promote collaborative efforts, develop a national quality measurement and reporting strategy, standardize health care performance measures, promote consumer understanding of quality information, and promote an enhanced system capacity for evaluation.

NOTE: JCAHO = Joint Commission on Accreditation of Healthcare Organizations; NCQA = National Committee for Quality Assurance; NQF = National Quality Forum.
SOURCES: AQA Alliance (2006); The Joint Commission (2007); NCQA (2007); NQF (2007).

know how a particular intervention is likely to affect patients with multiple comorbidities, such patients are frequently excluded from research studies and are often not covered by clinical guidelines (Boyd et al., 2005). In addition, relatively little is known about interventions for rare diseases

(European Organisation for Rare Diseases, 2005). Moreover, even though the evidence that is presented in systematic reviews may be comprehensive, it does not necessarily come in a form that is meaningful to doctors. For example, review documents typically summarize treatment effects in terms of relative risk, which does not take into account the prevalence of the disease. They also may not account for the presence of comorbidities. Physicians may prefer to make treatment decisions according to the absolute risks and benefits of treatment (presented as the number of events per 100 patients treated or the number of patients who need to be treated to prevent a single event) (Jackson and Feder, 1998).

Consumers also have unmet information needs. Direct-to-consumer advertising encourages greater spending on prescription drugs, which may potentially avert the underuse of medication but which may also promote medication overuse (Donohue et al., 2007). Consumers need to know when claims are valid and apply to them and when the claims are exaggerated or irrelevant to their needs. Physicians must be prepared to respond to consumer requests for information on heavily marketed prescription drugs and other clinical services, and they are also the target of aggressive sales efforts by pharmaceutical representatives (Angell, 2004).

Inconsistent Coding

The organizations that provide systematic reviews and clinical guidelines use different grading systems to characterize the quality of evidence and the strength of recommendations. These codes fall primarily into four categories: letters only (e.g., A, B, and C), Roman numerals only (e.g., I, II, and III), mixed letters and numerals (e.g., Ia, Ib, and IIa), and terms (e.g., strong and weak or consistent and inconsistent) (Schünemann et al., 2003). The discrepancies among grading systems cause difficulties for end users, who must decipher and remember what each of the various designations means. AHRQ identified more than 100 scales, checklists, and other instruments used to rate the quality of individual studies and the strength of bodies of evidence (AHRQ, 2002).

Transparency

Although by definition systematic reviews are supposed to use scientific methods to synthesize the available evidence, the organizations that produce these syntheses do not always make the processes and deliberations that they used public and transparent. Few organizations depend on an externally reviewed protocol to conduct their reviews. Consequently, the steps taken to address some of the difficult—often very subjective—elements of the synthesis process, such as the basis for including or excluding particular articles from reviews, are not apparent. Moher and colleagues (2007) assessed 300 systematic reviews and found that only 56 percent reported their full literature search strategy.

The same concerns apply to all evidence reviews, whether they are conducted by the various professional and advocacy groups or by government organizations. Whereas some groups closely adhere to evidence-based principles in supporting their clinical recommendations, many do not (Shaneyfelt et al., 1999). As a result, transparency is a key concern. One large study found that 87 percent of the clinical practice guidelines did not say whether a systematic search for published studies had been conducted (Grilli et al., 2000). Under those circumstances, users will have difficulty assuring themselves that the evidence is truly comprehensive or whether a subjective selection process has transpired. The lack of availability of transparent methods sections in evidence reviews reduces the ability of these users to make conscientious comparisons of guidelines addressing the same topic.

Financial Interests

A number of questions regarding the objectivity of organizations that develop practice guidelines have been raised. Professional societies, for example, may be subject to pressures from parts of their constituencies and individuals who have a substantial economic or professional stake in the intervention being considered, and these pressures have the potential to bias the guideline development process (Schwartz, 1984). Moreover, guideline development groups may receive funding from organizations affected by the findings, leading to concerns about the objectivity of their conclusions (Saul, 2006).

Panels supported by public-sector organizations, such as the FDA and the NIH, have also been criticized for including panelists with financial ties to the manufacturers whose products are affected by the decisions. For example, among the nine NIH panelists who produced guidelines recommending lower cholesterol targets in 2004, six had each received research grants, speaking honoraria, or consulting fees from at least three—and in some cases all five—of the statin manufacturers, which stood to profit from the decision. Only one panel member had no financial ties of some type to statin manufacturers (Kassirer, 2004). Recently, these concerns have led to the development of more restrictive conflict of interest measures at the FDA and the NIH (NIH, 2004; Vedantam, 2007).

Policy makers also become involved in decision making that is affected by private financial interests. One example is erythropoietin, an injectable drug used for the treatment of anemia in dialysis patients. In 2005, erythropoietin cost the Medicare program $1.75 billion—more than any other medication. The treatment of anemia focuses in part upon maintaining the level of hematocrit, a measure of red blood cell mass, within a target range. In 1989, the FDA established a recommended target hematocrit level of 30 to 33 percent. Under lobbying pressure from manufacturers, Congress encouraged CMS to broaden its payment policy, and in 2006 CMS allowed the target range to extend to 39 percent and above. This increase had a substantial impact on treatment utilization and cost. However, several studies showed that dialysis patients assigned to higher hematocrit target levels did not have better rates of survival, rates of hospitalization, or cardiac outcomes and in fact could be prone to adverse cardiovascular events, including myocardial infarction, vascular access thrombosis, increased use of antihypertensive medications, and cerebrovascular events (Cotter et al., 2006).

In a report released in 2007, the FDA indicated that it had found no evidence indicating that the anemia medicines improved quality of life or extended survival in cancer or dialysis patients. In fact, several studies suggested that the drugs can shorten patients' lives when they are used at high doses (Berenson and Pollack, 2007). A CMS coverage decision in 2007 stated that the evidence was sufficient to conclude that treatment with an erythropoiesis-stimulating agent is not reasonable and necessary for beneficiaries with certain clinical conditions, such as anemia associated with the treatment of leukemia (CMS, 2007a).

Unnecessary Duplications of Effort

In general, current efforts to assess clinical effectiveness are poorly coordinated, and there are significant duplications of effort (Hibble et al., 1998; Silagy et al., 2001; Timmermans and Mauck, 2005). Multiple stakeholders expend considerable resources essentially repeating work that has been done elsewhere or adding to that work. Frequently, the professional societies and payers that use evidence assessments as a basis for their decision making conduct their own supplementary evidence assessments if an existing synthesis is poorly done, not transparent, or out of date.

Many organizations may believe that they must review bodies of evidence—and often the same bodies of evidence—as part of their professional obligation. The list of organizations that add their voice is long and diverse: professional societies, individual physicians, health plans and purchasers, patients and consumer advocacy groups, producers of consumer decision aids, trade associations, manufacturers, public and private systematic reviewers, health services researchers, universities, think tanks, consultancy groups, Medicare contractors, federal regulators, NIH panels, state and federal policy makers, state and federal courts, and even the media. Not surprisingly, this often results in a cacophony of voices that in the aggregate is indecipherable and incongruent. When organizations replicate each other's work, they often expend resources that might have been better used to fill in other gaps in the knowledge base.

REFERENCES

Abramson, J. 2004. *Overdosed America: The broken promise of American medicine.* New York: HarperCollins Publishers.

ACC (American College of Cardiology). 2007. *ACC and performance measures* http://www.acc.org/qualityandscience/clinical/measures/intro.htm (accessed March 2, 2007).

ACP (American College of Physicians). 2007. *CEAP process* http://www.acponline.org/clinical/guidelines/ceap.htm (accessed March 12, 2007).

ADA (American Dietetic Association). 2007. *Evidence based practice* http://www.eatright.org/cps/rde/xchg/ada/hs.xsl/home_1075_ENU_HTML.htm (accessed March 12, 2007).

AHRQ (Agency for Healthcare Research and Quality). 2001. *Improving the health and health care of older Americans.* Rockville, MD: AHRQ.

———. 2002. *Fact sheet: Rating the strength of scientific research findings.* Rockville, MD: AHRQ.

———. 2007a. *About USPSTF* http://www.ahrq.gov/clinic/uspstfab.htm (accessed March 2, 2007).

———. 2007b. *Effective Health Care Program—About us* http://effectivehealthcare.ahrq.gov/aboutUs/index.cfm (accessed September 12, 2007).

———. 2007c. *Evidence-based Practice Centers* http://www.ahrq.gov/clinic/epc/ (accessed March 2, 2007).

Altman, D. E., and L. Levitt. 2002. The sad history of health care cost containment as told in one chart. *Health Affairs* w2.83.

America's Health Insurance Plans. 2007. *Setting a higher bar: We believe there is more the nation can do to improve quality and safety in health care.* Washington, DC: America's Health Insurance Plans.

American Diabetes Association. 2007. *Clinical practice recommendations* http://www.diabetes.org/for-health-professionals-and-scientists/cpr.jsp (accessed March 12, 2007).

Angell, M. 2004. *The truth about the drug companies: How they deceive us and what to do about it.* New York: Random House.

AQA Alliance. 2006. *AQA Background: Improving clinical quality and consumer decision-making* http://www.aqaalliance.org/files/Backgrounddocument.doc (accessed March 12, 2007).

ASCO (American Society of Clinical Oncology). 2007. *Quality care & guidelines* http://www.asco.org/portal/site/ASCO/menuitem.56bbfed7341ace64e7cba5b4320041a0/?vgnextoid=38e748fa20e3e010VgnVCM100000ed730ad1RCRD&vgnextfmt=default (accessed March 12, 2007).

Atkins, D., K. Fink, and J. Slutsky. 2005a. Better information for better health care: The Evidence-based Practice Center program and the Agency for Healthcare Research and Quality. *Annals of Internal Medicine* 142(12):1035-1041.

Atkins, D., J. Siegel, and J. Slutsky. 2005b. Making policy when the evidence is in dispute. *Health Affairs* 24(1):102-113.

Baicker, K., K. S. Buckles, and A. Chandra. 2006. Geographic variation in the appropriate use of cesarean delivery. *Health Affairs* 25(5):w355-w367.

BCBSA (Blue Cross and Blue Shield Association). 2007a. *Blue Cross and Blue Shield Association proposes payer-funded institute to evaluate what medical treatments work best* http://www.bcbs.com/news/bcbsa/blue-cross-and-blue-shield-association-proposes-payer-funded-institute.html (accessed May 2007).

————. 2007b. *Technology Evaluation Center* http://www.bcbs.com/betterknowledge/tec/ (accessed March 2, 2007).

Berenson, A., and A. Pollack. 2007. Doctors reap millions for anemia drugs. *The New York Times* http://www.nytimes.com/2007/05/09/business/09anemia.html?ex=1186804800& en=c43b43ab957a82e5&ei=5070 (accessed May 9, 2007).

Bergthold, L. A. 1995. Medical necessity: Do we need it? *Health Affairs* 14(4):180-190.

Berwick, D. M., N.-A. DeParle, D. M. Eddy, P. M. Ellwood, A. C. Enthoven, G. C. Halvorson, K. W. Kizer, E. A. McGlynn, U. E. Reinhardt, R. D. Reischauer, W. L. Roper, J. W. Rowe, L. D. Schaeffer, J. E. Wennberg, and G. R. Wilensky. 2003. Paying for performance: Medicare should lead. *Health Affairs* 22(6):8-10.

Borger, C., S. Smith, C. Truffer, S. Keehan, A. Sisko, J. Poisal, and M. K. Clemens. 2006. Health spending projections through 2015: Changes on the horizon. *Health Affairs* 25(2):w61-w73.

Boyd, C. M., J. Darer, C. Boult, L. P. Fried, L. Boult, and A. W. Wu. 2005. Clinical practice guidelines and quality of care for older patients with multiple comorbid diseases: Implications for pay for performance. *JAMA* 294(6):716-724.

Buntin, M. B., C. Damberg, A. Haviland, K. Kapur, N. Lurie, R. McDevitt, and M. S. Marquis. 2006. Consumer-directed health care: Early evidence about effects on cost and quality. *Health Affairs* 25(6):w516-w530.

CDER (Center for Drug Evaluation and Research). 2007. *The CDER handbook* http://www. fda.gov/cder/handbook/index.htm (accessed August 1, 2007).

Clancy, C. M. 2003. *Testimony on technology, innovation, and the costs of health care before the Joint Economic Committee.* Rockville, MD: AHRQ.

CMS (Centers for Medicare & Medicaid Services). 2006. *Factors CMS considers in referring topics to the Medicare Evidence Development & Coverage Advisory Committee* http:// www.cms.hhs.gov/mcd/ncpc_view_document.asp?id=10 (accessed August 12, 2007).

————. 2007a. *Decision memo for Erythropoiesis Stimulating Agents (ESAs) for non-renal disease indications (CAG-00383N)* https://www.cms.hhs.gov/mcd/viewdecisionmemo. asp?id=203 (accessed August 17, 2007).

————. 2007b. *Medicare Evidence Development & Coverage Advisory Committee* http:// www.cms.hhs.gov/FACA/02_MedCAC.asp#TopOfPage (accessed March 2, 2007).

Cochrane Collaboration. 2007. *About us* http://www.cochrane.org/docs/descrip.htm (accessed July 12, 2007).

Congressional Budget Office. 2006. *Consumer-directed health plans: Potential effects on health care spending and outcomes* http://www.cbo.gov/ftpdocs/77xx/doc7700/12-21-HealthPlans.pdf (accessed July 11, 2007).

————. 2007. Research on the comparative effectiveness of medical treatments: Options for an expanded federal role. *Testimony by Director Peter R. Orszag before House Ways and Means Subcommittee on Health* http://www.cbo.gov/ftpdocs/82xx/doc8209/ Comparative_Testimony.pdf (accessed June 12, 2007).

Cotter, D., M. Thamer, K. Narasimhan, Y. Zhang, and K. Bullock. 2006. Translating epoetin research into practice: The role of government and the use of scientific evidence. *Health Affairs* 25(5):1249-1259.

Cutler, D. M. 2005. The potential for cost savings in Medicare's future. *Health Affairs* w5.r77.

Cutler, D. M., and M. McClellan. 2001. Is technological change in medicine worth it? *Health Affairs* 20(5):11-29.

The Dartmouth Atlas Project. 2003 (unpublished). *Medicare spending per capita in the United States, by hospital referral region.* Dartmouth College, New Hampshire.

DERP (Drug Effectiveness Review Project). 2007. *Description* http://www.ohsu.edu/ drugeffectiveness/description/index.htm (accessed March 2, 2007).

Donohue, J. M., M. Cevasco, and M. B. Rosenthal. 2007. A decade of direct-to-consumer advertising of prescription drugs. *New England Journal of Medicine* 357(7):673-681.

Druss, B. G., and S. C. Marcus. 2005. Growth and decentralization of the medical literature: Implications for evidence-based medicine. *Journal of the Medical Library Association* 93(4):499-501.

Eagle, K. A., and R. A. Guyton. 2004. *ACC/AHA 2004 Guideline update for coronary artery bypass graft surgery.* Bethesda, MD: American College of Cardiology/American Heart Association Task Force on Practice Guidelines.

ECRI Institute. 2007. *About ECRI Institute* http://www.ecri.org/About/Pages/default.aspx (accessed March 2, 2007).

European Organisation for Rare Diseases. 2005. *Rare diseases: Understanding this public health priority.* Paris: European Organisation for Rare Diseases.

Feenberg, D., and J. Skinner. 2000. Federal transfers across states: Winners and losers. *National Tax Journal* 53(3 Part 2):713-732.

Fisher, E. S., D. E. Wennberg, T. A. Stukel, D. J. Gottlieb, F. L. Lucas, and E. L. Pinder. 2003a. The implications of regional variations in Medicare spending. Part 1: The content, quality, and accessibility of care. *Annals of Internal Medicine* 138(4):273-287.

———. 2003b. The implications of regional variations in Medicare Spending. Part 2: Health outcomes and satisfaction with care. *Annals of Internal Medicine* 138(4):288-298.

Fuchs, V. R. 2004. Perspective: More variation in use of case, more flat-of-the-curve medicine. *Health Affairs* 104.

Garber, A. M. 2001. Evidence-based coverage policy. *Health Affairs* 20(5):62-82.

Gelijns, A., and N. Rosenberg. 1994. The dynamics of technological change in medicine. *Health Affairs* 13(3):28-46.

Grilli, R., N. Magrini, A. Penna, G. Mura, and A. Liberati. 2000. Practice guidelines developed by specialty societies: The need for critical appraisal. *Lancet* 355:103-106.

Guadagnoli, E., P. J. Hauptman, J. Z. Ayanian, C. L. Pashos, B. J. McNeil, and P. D. Cleary. 1995. Variation in the use of cardiac procedures after acute myocardial infarction. *New England Journal of Medicine* 333(9):573-578.

Hayes, Inc. 2007. *About us* http://www.hayesinc.com/aboutus/ (accessed March 2, 2007).

The Henry J. Kaiser Family Foundation. 2007. *Medicare: A primer.* Washington, DC: The Henry J. Kaiser Family Foundation.

Hibble, A., D. Kanka, D. Pencheon, and F. Pooles. 1998. Guidelines in general practice: The new Tower of Babel? *BMJ* 317(7162):862-863.

Iglehart, J. K. 2001. America's love affair with medical innovation. *Health Affairs* 20(5):6-7.

IOM (Institute of Medicine). 2001. *Crossing the quality chasm: A new health system for the 21st century.* Washington, DC: National Academy Press.

———. 2003. *Unequal treatment: Confronting racial and ethnic disparities in health care.* Edited by Smedley, B. D., A. Y. Stith, and A. R. Nelson. Washington, DC: The National Academies Press.

———. 2007a. *Learning what works best: The nation's need for evidence on comparative effectiveness in health care* http://www.iom.edu/ebm-effectiveness (accessed April 2007).

———. 2007b. *Rewarding provider performance: Aligning incentives in Medicare, pathways to quality health care series.* Washington, DC: The National Academies Press.

Jackson, R., and G. Feder. 1998. Guidelines for clinical guidelines. *BMJ* 317(7156):427-428.

The Joint Commission. 2007. *Facts about the Joint Commission* http://www.jointcommission.org/AboutUs/joint_commission_facts.htm (accessed March 12, 2007).

Joint Economic Committee. 2007. *Nanotechnology: The future is coming sooner than you think.* Washington, DC: United States Congress.

Kassirer, J. P. 2004. Why should we swallow what these studies say? *The Washington Post*, B03, http://www.washingtonpost.com/wp-dyn/articles/A29456-2004Jul31.html (accessed July 2007).

Loscalzo, J. 2006. The NIH budget and the future of biomedical research. *New England Journal of Medicine* 354(16):1665-1667.

Lubitz, J. 2005. Health, technology, and medical care spending. *Health Affairs* w5.r81.

Meadows, M. 2005. Genomics and personalized medicine. *FDA Consumer Magazine* November/December.

Medicare Payment Advisory Commission. 2007. Chapter 2: Producing comparative effectiveness information. In *Report to the Congress: Promoting greater efficiency in Medicare* http://www.medpac.gov/documents/Jun07_EntireReport.pdf (accessed June 2007).

Mitka, M. 2004. Is PSA testing still useful? *JAMA* 292(19):2326-2327.

Moher, D., J. Tetzlaff, A. C. Tricco, M. Sampson, and D. G. Altman. 2007. Epidemiology and reporting characteristics of systematic reviews. *PLoS Medicine* 4(3):447-455.

NCQA (National Committee for Quality Assurance). 2007. *About NCQA* http://web.ncqa.org/tabid/65/Default.aspx (accessed March 12, 2007).

Neumann, P. J., and E. A. Sandberg. 1998. Trends in health care R&D and technology innovation. *Health Affairs* 17(6):111-119.

NGC (National Guideline Clearinghouse). 2007a. *Guideline index* http://www.guideline.gov/browse/guideline_index.aspx (accessed September 14, 2007).

———. 2007b. *Search for antihypertensives* http://www.guideline.gov/search/searchresults.aspx?Type=3&txtSearch=antihypertensives&num=20 (accessed July 11, 2007).

NHLBI (National Heart, Lung, and Blood Institute). 2007. *Information for health professionals . . . clinical practice guidelines* http://www.nhlbi.nih.gov/guidelines/index.htm (accessed November 15, 2007).

NIH (National Institutes of Health). 2004. *Report of the National Institutes of Health Blue Ribbon Panel on Conflict of Interest Policies June 22, 2004*. Washington, DC: NIH.

NIH Consensus Development Program. 2007. *About us* http://consensus.nih.gov/ABOUTCDP.htm (accessed April 8, 2007).

NQF (National Quality Forum). 2007. *About us* http://www.qualityforum.org/about/ (accessed March 12, 2007).

PhRMA. 2006. R&D investments by America's pharmaceutical research companies near record $40 billion in 2005. *Press Release* http://www.phrma.org/news_room/press_releases/r%26d_investments_by_america%92s_pharmaceutical_research_companies_nears_record_%2440_billion_in_2005/ (accessed September 12, 2007).

Redberg, R. F. 2007. Evidence, appropriateness, and technology assessment in cardiology: A case study of computed tomography. *Health Affairs* 26(1):86-95.

Saul, S. 2006. Unease on industry's role in hypertension debate. *The New York Times*. May 20.

Schünemann, H. J., D. Best, G. Vist, A. D. Oxman, and the GRADE Working Group. 2003. Letters, numbers, symbols and words: How to communicate grades of evidence and recommendations. *Canadian Medical Association Journal* 169(7):677-680.

Schwartz, J. S. 1984. The role of professional medical societies in reducing practice variations. *Health Affairs* 3(2):90-101.

Shaneyfelt, T. M., M. F. Mayo-Smith, and J. Rothwangl. 1999. Are guidelines following guidelines?: The methodological quality of clinical practice guidelines in the peer-reviewed medical literature. *JAMA* 281(20):1900-1905.

Shortell, S. M., T. G. Rundall, and J. Hsu. 2007. Improving patient care by linking evidence-based medicine and evidence-based management. *JAMA* 298(6):673-676.

Silagy, C. A., L. F. Stead, and T. Lancaster. 2001. Use of systematic reviews in clinical practice guidelines: Case study of smoking cessation. *BMJ* 323(7317):833-836.

Skinner, J., and J. E. Wennberg. 2003. Perspective: Exceptionalism or extravagance? What's different about health care in south Florida? *Health Affairs* w3.372.

Sung, N. S., W. F. Crowley, Jr., M. Genel, P. Salber, L. Sandy, L. M. Sherwood, S. B. Johnson, V. Catanese, H. Tilson, K. Getz, E. L. Larson, D. Scheinberg, E. A. Reece, H. Slavkin, A. Dobs, J. Grebb, R. A. Martinez, A. Korn, and D. Rimoin. 2003. Central challenges facing the national clinical research enterprise. *JAMA* 289(10):1278-1287.

Timmermans, S., and A. Mauck. 2005. The promises and pitfalls of evidence-based medicine. *Health Affairs* 24(1):18-28.

Tunis, S. R. 2005. A clinical research strategy to support shared decision making. *Health Affairs* 24(1):180-184.

Tunis, S. R., and S. D. Pearson. 2006. Coverage options for promising technologies: Medicare's "Coverage with evidence development." *Health Affairs* 25(5):1218-1230.

Tunis, S. R., D. B. Stryer, and C. M. Clancy. 2003. Practical clinical trials: Increasing the value of clinical research for decision making in clinical and health policy. *JAMA* 290(12): 1624-1632.

U.S. Government Accountability Office. 2006. *Consumer-directed health plans: Small but growing enrollment fueled by rising cost of health care coverage.* GAO-06-514. Washington, DC: Government Printing Office.

———. 2007. *State and local governments: Persistent fiscal challenges will likely emerge within the next decade.* GAO-07-1080SP. Washington, DC: Government Printing Office.

Vedantam, S. 2007. FDA moves to try to reduce conflicts of interest on boards. *The Washington Post*, A12, http://www.washingtonpost.com/wp-dyn/content/article/2007/03/21/AR2007032102068.html (accessed September 12, 2007).

Walker, D. 2007. Long term budget outlook: Saving our future requires tough choices today. In *U.S. Senate Budget Committee*. Washington, DC: General Accounting Office.

Walsh, G. 2005. Biopharmaceuticals: Recent approvals and likely directions. *Trends in Biotechnology* 23(11):553-558.

Weinstein, J. N., K. K. Bronner, T. S. Morgan, and J. E. Wennberg. 2004. Trends and geographic variations in major surgery for degenerative diseases of the hip, knee, and spine. *Health Affairs* var.81.

Wennberg, J. E. 1988. Improving the medical decision-making process. *Health Affairs* 7(1): 99-106.

———. 2004. Perspective: Practice variations and health care reform: Connecting the dots. *Health Affairs* var.140.

Wennberg, D. E., and J. E. Wennberg. 2003. Perspective: Addressing variations: Is there hope for the future? *Health Affairs* w3.614.

Wennberg, J. E., E. S. Fisher, and J. S. Skinner. 2002a. Geography and the debate over Medicare reform. *Health Affairs* Jul-Dec (Suppl Web Exclusives):w96-w114.

———. 2002b. Geography and the debate over Medicare reform. *Health Affairs* w2.96.

Wennberg, J. E., E. S. Fisher, T. A. Stukel, and S. M. Sharp. 2004. Use of Medicare claims data to monitor provider-specific performance among patients with severe chronic illness. *Health Affairs* var.5.

Wennberg, J. E., E. S. Fisher, and S. M. Sharp. 2006. *The care of patients with severe chronic illness.* Lebanon, NH: The Dartmouth Atlas of Health Care.

Wilensky, G. R. 2006. Developing a center for comparative effectiveness information. *Health Affairs* 25(6):w572-w585.

Windish, D. M., S. J. Huot, and M. L. Green. 2007. Medicine residents' understanding of the biostatistics and results in the medical literature. *JAMA* 298(9):1010-1022.

Zinner, D. E. 2001. Medical R&D at the turn of the millennium. *Health Affairs* 20(5): 202-209.

3

Setting Priorities for
Evidence Assessment

Abstract: This chapter provides the committee's findings and recommendations on setting priorities for evidence assessment (systematic review) and describes key challenges in establishing a priority setting process for a national clinical assessment program ("the Program"). The committee recommends that the Program appoint an independent, standing Priority Setting Advisory Committee (PSAC) to develop and implement the process. PSAC members should be selected to ensure a balance of expertise and interests, with minimal bias due to conflicts of interest. Although there is little solid basis to recommend the use of one priority setting process over another, the committee recommends that the process adhere to basic principles of consistency, efficiency, objectivity, responsiveness, and transparency. Thus, the PSAC should establish a process that is open, predictable, and explicitly defined, with fully documented standards and procedures. The procedures should be simple and efficient to preserve the available resources for evidence assessment itself. Two considerations should be paramount in identifying the highest priority topics: (1) how well the topic reflects the clinical questions of patients and clinicians and (2) the potential for the topics to have a strong impact on clinical and other outcomes that matter the most to patients.

If the nation is to resolve the current deficiencies in how it uses scientific evidence to identify the most effective clinical services, there must be a process for identifying the most important topics in order to preserve resources for evidence assessment itself. Most health technology assessment programs have an organized process for determining which topics merit comprehensive study. At present, however, no one agency or organization in the United States evaluates from a broad, national perspective the effectiveness of new as well as established health interventions for all populations, children as well as elderly people, women as well as men, and ethnic and racial minorities.

As noted in Chapter 1, this report focuses on developing an organizational framework for a national clinical effectiveness assessment program, referred throughout as "the Program." Early in its deliberations, the committee agreed that the Program should commission systematic reviews on the effectiveness of health services and that the topics of the reviews should be informed by the recommendations of an independent Priority Setting Advisory Committee (PSAC). The objective of this chapter is threefold: (1) to review the basic elements of a priority setting process, (2) to present the committee's recommendations for establishing a priority setting infrastructure, and (3) to highlight key programmatic challenges in establishing a priority setting process for the Program.

> **Recommendation: The Program should appoint a standing Priority Setting Advisory Committee to identify high-priority topics for systematic reviews of clinical effectiveness.**

BACKGROUND

This section provides background on the basic elements of a priority setting process: identifying potential topics, selecting the priority criteria, reducing the initial list of nominated topics to a smaller set of topics to be pursued, and choosing the final priority topics. Some approaches also incorporate quantitative methods that involve the collection of data that can be used to weigh priorities, the assignment of scores for each criterion to each topic, and the calculation of priority scores for each topic to produce a ranked priority list. A committee or advisory group that reviews and chooses the topics that will be funded typically conducts the process. It may use a formal method, such as the Delphi technique, to systematically develop the high-priority list. The Delphi technique has been adapted and modified in various ways to facilitate group decision making (OTA, 1994). It typically involves the distribution of a questionnaire to an expert group. Each participant independently answers the questionnaires. The responses are summarized and reported back to the group. The process may be anonymous or open, and several iterations may be necessary before a final decision is reached.

What Is the Best Approach?

No single priority setting method is obviously superior to others (Goodman, 2004; Noorani et al., 2007; Oxman et al., 2006; Sassi, 2003). The committee could not find any systematic assessments of the comparative strengths and weaknesses of different approaches to priority setting, including whether complex quantitative and resource-intensive methods are more effective than less rigorous approaches.

Apparently, few, if any, organizations use a quantitative approach to selecting priority topics, although numerous methods have been developed. Phelps and Parente (1990), for example, developed a formula for calculating a priority index for health technology assessment. The Institute of Medicine (IOM) Committee on Priorities for Assessment and Reassessment of Health Care Technologies proposed a method that could be used to aggregate various dimensions into a single priority score, including a technique that quantifies the potential gains that can achieved by assessing health interventions (IOM, 1992).[1]

Various Contexts for Setting Priorities

Organizations have different objectives and target audiences for evidence assessment. The annual number of selected topics that are reviewed is quite small (Table 3-1). In 2006, for example, the number of systematic reviews produced by federal agencies ranged from only 3 by the National Institutes of Health (NIH) Consensus Development Program to 22 by the Agency for Healthcare Research and Quality (AHRQ) Evidence-based Practice Centers (EPCs). There are no aggregate national data on the volume of topics that are assessed each year.

The range of potential topics that may be considered may include the universe of prevention such as screening tests or immunizations, diagnosis such as laboratory tests or imaging techniques, drugs and other therapeutic interventions such as surgery, chemotherapy, or radiation, and end-of-life care and palliation. However, the specific audience for the assessment is likely to have more narrow interests, such as new and emerging technologies or a specific subpopulation group. For example, the Blue Cross and Blue Shield Association (BCBSA) Technology Evaluation Center (TEC) focuses on the specific needs of member plans. The Medicare Evidence Development and Coverage Advisory Committee (MedCAC), which advises

---

[1]See the following IOM reports for past recommendations related to priority setting: *Setting Priorities for Health Technologies Assessment: A Model Process* (IOM, 1992), *Setting Priorities for Clinical Practice Guidelines* (IOM, 1995), *National Priorities for the Assessment of Clinical Conditions and Medical Technologies: Report of a Pilot Study* (IOM, 1990), and *Priority Areas for National Action: Transforming Health Care Quality* (IOM, 2003).

TABLE 3-1 Context for Setting Priorities for Evidence Assessment, 2006

Organization	Target Audience	Number of Full Systematic Reviews
AHRQ		
Effective Heath Care Program	CMS, providers, policy makers, consumers	4
EPC program	CMS, USPSTF, NIH, and other federal agencies; providers; medical professional societies	22
USPSTF	Primary care clinicians, health systems, payers, and purchasers	6
Other federal programs		
CMS	Medicare intermediaries, beneficiaries, and providers	9
DERP	State Medicaid programs	3
NIH Consensus Development Program	Health professionals and the public	3
Private technology assessors		
BCBSA TEC	Medical directors of BCBSA member plans, providers, and scientific staff	14
ECRI Institute	Private clients, including decision makers in hospitals, health systems, health plans, and departments and ministries of health	20
Hayes, Inc.	Private clients, including decision makers in hospitals, health systems, health plans, and government agencies	86

NOTE: DERP = Drug Effectiveness Review Project; USPSTF = U.S. Preventive Services Task Force.
SOURCES: AHRQ (2007c,d,e); BCBSA TEC (2007); NIH Consensus Development Program (2007).

the Centers for Medicare & Medicaid Services (CMS) on the services used by the Medicare population, sponsors evidence reviews (conducted by an AHRQ EPC) only when Medicare is considering a national coverage decision on a controversial issue.

In general, payers initiate assessments when they must make benefits and coverage decisions about new technologies or new applications of existing technologies. In this context, the decision usually involves a categorical determination (e.g., are insulin pumps covered?) or a more narrow assessment to identify the subpopulations for which a service should be covered (e.g., who among the population is likely to benefit from an artificial disc for degenerative disc disease?). If the topic in question is not within the boundaries of covered benefits, payers are unlikely to assess it. Thus, for example, an insurance company is not likely to assess the efficacy of a vaccine if it does not cover preventive services.

The agenda of AHRQ, the lead federal health agency charged with conducting systematic reviews of clinical effectiveness, is circumscribed by statute. The Effective Health Care Program, for example, may only sponsor studies related to 1 of 10 priority conditions established by the secretary of the U.S. Department of Health and Human Services (Table 3-2). The U.S. Preventive Services Task Force (USPSTF) focuses on clinical preventive services provided in primary care settings. Many medical professional societies assess evidence to develop clinical guidelines for the management of specific conditions. Manufacturers assess evidence to demonstrate safety and efficacy and to persuade payers and other constituencies of their value. Private research firms generally focus on responding to marketplace demands.

The Cochrane Collaboration supports the broadest range of evidence reviews worldwide; its volunteer researchers participate in 51 discipline-specific (e.g., musculoskeletal) review groups that set their own agendas in accord with the important questions within their disciplines. The Cochrane Collaboration's Steering Group is considering new approaches to how the review groups set priorities for their research and has funded research projects whose results will guide them in this effort (Cochrane Collaboration, 2007).

Methods Used to Identify Potential Topics

Some organizations, including AHRQ and the USPSTF, actively solicit nominations from stakeholders and the public (Table 3-2). Other organizations have internal processes for gathering suggestions from staff or outside advisors.

The response to the AHRQ open call for topics is of interest, although it is not necessarily indicative of the potential response to a broader call for topics from a well-funded agency. Table 3-3 shows the number of EPC topics nominated and funded, the topic areas, and the types of organizations that nominated a topic for the EPC program during 2005 and 2006. The total number of nominations was small. From 2005 to 2006, AHRQ received 76 topic nominations: 36 were related to treatment effectiveness; 13 were related to diagnostic interventions; and the rest concerned quality improvement and patient safety, prevention, organization and finance, and other topics. Ultimately, 51 percent of the topics were funded.

TABLE 3-2 Methods Used to Identify Topics for Systematic Reviews in Selected Organizations

Organization	Methods	Who Can Nominate	Eligible Topics
AHRQ	Solicits topics annually through the *Federal Register* and accepts nominations on an ongoing basis	Open to the public; AHRQ conducts systematic reviews for CMS, the USPSTF, and the NIH Consensus Development Conference program	Effectiveness of prevention, diagnosis, treatment, and management of common clinical and behavioral conditions; organization and financing; and research methods; topics addressed by the Effective Health Care Program must relate to 1 of 10 priority conditions established by the secretary of HHS[a]
BCBSA TEC	Solicits topics from within BCBSA and from its advisers	TEC staff, medical directors of member plans, Medical Advisory Panel (external advisers), Medical Policy Panel, and pharmacy managers	Effectiveness of surgical procedures, devices and implants, diagnostic imaging, laboratory tests, and targeted and specialty pharmaceuticals
Cochrane Collaboration	Vary among 51 review groups	Open to the public; reviews are author initiated or the topic is nominated and authors sought	Broad range of clinical services and population-based health interventions
DERP[b]	Program participants nominate topics	State Medicaid programs and other participating organizations	Comparative effectiveness of drugs within classes of drugs
MedCAC and CMS[b]	Internal decision	MedCAC staff	Devices, drugs, and procedures that are within the scope of Medicare coverage and subject to a national coverage decision
NICE	Internal decision by the department of health in England and Wales; NICE uses the National Horizon Scanning Centre to identify new and emerging technologies	Individuals and groups	Effectiveness of services that are being considered for coverage by the National Health Service, including drugs, devices, diagnostics, surgical procedures, and population-based health promotion

TABLE 3-2 Continued

Organization	Methods	Who Can Nominate	Eligible Topics
NIH OMAR[b]	NIH institutes and centers and OMAR select topics on the basis of four criteria	NIH institutes and centers, the U.S. Congress, other government health agencies, and the public	Medical safety and efficacy; economic, sociological, legal, and ethical issues
USPSTF[b]	Solicits topics biennially through the *Federal Register* and appeals to stakeholders	Open to the public	Clinical preventive services, including screening, counseling, and preventive medications for asymptomatic individuals

NOTE: DERP = Drug Effectiveness Review Project; HHS = U.S. Department of Health and Human Services; NICE = National Institute for Health and Clinical Excellence; NIH OMAR = National Institutes of Health Office of Medical Applications of Research.

[a]The priority conditions are arthritis and nontraumatic joint disorders, cancer, chronic obstructive pulmonary disease and asthma, dementia, depression and other mood disorders, diabetes mellitus, ischemic heart disease, peptic ulcer disease and dyspepsia, pneumonia, and stroke and hypertension.

[b]The reviews are conducted by an AHRQ EPC.

SOURCES: AHRQ (2006, 2007b); Aronson (2007); Coates (2007); Cochrane Collaboration (2007); Guirguis-Blake et al. (2007); NIH Consensus Development Program (2005).

Box 3-1 lists the organizations that submitted EPC topic nominations from 2005 to 2006. The largest source of nominations was federal agencies, followed by medical professional societies (to support clinical guideline development). Box 3-2 provides the topics of EPC studies released during the same period; they include the diagnosis and treatment of cancer and blood disorders, heart and vascular diseases, mental health conditions, and neurological disorders; routine obstetric care; bioterrorism preparedness; the use of dietary supplements for various clinical conditions; information technology; research methodologies; and approaches to improving the quality and the safety of care.

Horizon Scanning

Many organizations, especially health plans and the private technology assessment firms that serve them, make special efforts to identify new or emerging technologies before they are widely adopted in practice. These activities, commonly referred to as "horizon scanning," typically involve the active monitoring of medical journals; trade press publications; national

TABLE 3-3 AHRQ EPC Study Nominations by Source and Topic Area, 2005-2006

Source or Topic Area	Number		Total	
	2005	2006	Number	Percent
All nominations	40	36	76	100.0
Funded nominations	24	15	39	51.3
Source (*n* = 47)				
Federal agencies	15	5	20	42.6
Health plans	2	1	3	6.4
Medical professional societies	10	6	16	34.0
Other	4	4	8	17.0
Total	31	16	47	100.0
Topic area (*n* = 76)				
Prevention	3	4	7	9.2
Diagnosis	5	8	13	17.1
Treatment	17	19	36	47.4
Rehabilitation	0	1	1	1.3
Organization and finance	2	4	6	7.9
Quality improvement and patient safety	8	0	8	10.5
Other	5	0	5	6.6

NOTE: Excludes studies requested by CMS and USPSTF.
SOURCE: Personal communication, J. Slutsky, Agency for Healthcare Research and Quality, May 10, 2007.

health news sources; CMS and U.S. Food and Drug Administration notices; announcements of proposed and new current procedural terminology codes; and abstracts, posters, and presentations from scientific meetings of major specialty societies for topics. There is no evidence or apparent consensus on the elements of an effective horizon-scanning system (Murphy et al., 2007).

Nevertheless, past experience has shown, sometimes with tragic consequences, the risks of failing to assess new and emerging health technologies before they are widely adopted. Although it is not clear that early effectiveness assessment would deter the rapid adoption of unproven interventions, assessments of the early evidence could underscore the risks of early adoption. A compelling example of what can go horribly wrong when a high-risk, untested procedure is promoted is high-dose chemotherapy with autologous bone marrow transplantation (HDC/ABMT) for breast cancer. Rettig and colleagues (2007) showed in an in-depth history of HDC/ABMT that no central entity required that the controversial new procedure be adequately evaluated before its use became widespread. At the time that HDC/ABMT began to be used, its potential risks and benefits were not known. With this void as the backdrop, the procedure was evaluated not by parties with the appropriate clinical or research expertise, but by the

---

BOX 3-1
Sources of Topic Nominations,
Evidence-based Practice Centers, 2005-2006

America's Health Insurance Plans
American Academy of Audiology
American Academy of Family Physicians
American Academy of Orthopedic Surgeons
American Academy of Pediatrics
American Association of Clinical Chemistry
American College of Cardiology
American College of Chest Physicians
American College of Obstetricians and Gynecologists
American College of Physicians
American Dental Association
American Dietetic Association
American Organization of Nurse Executives
American Society of Clinical Oncology
Centers for Disease Control and Prevention
Centers for Medicare & Medicaid Services
Council of Linkages Between Academia and Public Health Practice (Public Health
    Foundation)
Employer Health Care Alliance Cooperative
Fogarty International Center for Advanced Study in the Health Sciences (NIH)
Health Resources and Services Administration
National Center of Complementary and Alternative Medicine (NIH)
National Rural Health Association
Office of Dietary Supplements (NIH)
Office of Management Analysis and Review (NIH)
Office of Research on Women's Health (NIH)
Saliba Burns Institute
Society of Vascular Surgery
Spinal Cord Consortium
Transatlantic Inter-Society Consensus
Union County Health Committee
U.S. Breastfeeding Committee
U.S. Preventive Services Task Force

SOURCE: Personal Communication, J. Slutsky, Agency for Healthcare Research and Quality,
May 10, 2007.

---

courts, legislatures, and the media. Many women died of treatment-related causes before it was clear that HDC/ABMT was ineffective and harmful. Box 3-3 provides a number of examples of widely adopted health interventions found to be ineffective or harmful.

BOX 3-2
Topics of Evidence-based Practice
Center Reports, 2005 to present

Bioterrorism
  Pediatric Anthrax, Bioterrorism Preparedness
Cancer and blood disorders
  Adnexal Mass
  Cancer Care Quality Measures, Colorectal Cancer
  Cancer Care Quality Measures, Symptoms and End-of-Life
  Cancer Clinical Trials, Recruitment of Underrepresented Populations
  Hereditary Nonpolyposis Colorectal Cancer
  Ovarian Cancer, Genomic Tests for Detection and Management
  Small Cell Lung Cancer, Management
Complementary and alternative care
  Meditation Practices for Health
Dietary supplements
  B Vitamins and Berries and Age-Related Neurodegenerative Disorders
  Multivitamin/Mineral Supplements, Chronic Disease Prevention
  Omega-3 Fatty Acids Series: Effects on Cancer, Child and Maternal Health,
    Cognitive Functions, Eye Health, Mental Health, Organ Transplantation
  Soy, Effects on Health Outcomes
Ear, nose, and throat conditions
  Sinusitis, Acute Bacterial—Update
Heart and vascular diseases
  Abdominal Aortic Aneurysm, Endovascular and Open Surgical Repairs
  Heart Failure Diagnosis and Prognosis, Testing for BNP and NT-proBNP
  Left Ventricular Systolic Dysfunction, Cardiac Resynchronization Therapy and
    ICDs
  Post-Myocardial Infarction Depression
Information technology
  Health Information Technology, Costs and Benefits
  Telemedicine for the Medicare Population—Update
Lung conditions
  Asthma, Work-Related
  Chronic Obstructive Pulmonary Disease, Spirometry
Mental health conditions and substance abuse
  Adults with Non-Psychotic Depression Treated with SSRIs, CYP450 Testing
  Eating Disorders, Management
  Tobacco Use: Prevention, Cessation, and Control

The emphasis on horizon scanning appears to have led to a considerable duplication of effort among health plans and private technology assessment firms in the United States. In response to a request by the committee, UnitedHealthcare provided a sample list of the screening, diagnostic, therapeutic, and disease management services and devices that it had

Metabolic, nutritional, and endocrine conditions
Impaired Glucose Tolerance and Fasting Glucose, Diagnosis, Prognosis, and Therapy

Methodology
Empirical Evaluation, Association Between Methodological Shortcomings and Estimates of Adverse Events
Health Benefit Design, Consumer-Oriented Strategies for Improving
Statement of Work for Technical Analysis, Methodology
Systematic Reviews, Criteria for Distinguishing Effectiveness from Efficacy Trials

Nerve and brain conditions
Age-Related Neurodegenerative Disorders, B Vitamins and Berries
Insomnia, Manifestations and Management
Stroke, Evaluation and Treatment

Obstetric and gynecologic conditions
Breastfeeding, Maternal and Infant Health Outcomes
Cesarean Delivery on Maternal Request
Episiotomy Use in Obstetrical Care
Menopause-Related Symptoms, Management
Ovarian Cancer, Genomic Tests for Detection and Management
Perinatal Depression: Prevalence and Screening
Uterine Fibroids—Update

Pediatric conditions
Breastfeeding, Maternal and Infant Health Outcomes
Toilet Training, Effectiveness of Different Methods

Quality improvement and patient safety
Children with Special Health Care Needs, Care Coordination Strategies
Closing the Quality Gap—Vol. 3: Hypertension Care; Vol. 4: Antibiotic Prescribing Behavior; Vol. 5: Asthma Care, Vol. 6: Healthcare-Associated Infections; Vol. 7: Care Coordination
Continuing Medical Education, Effectiveness
Nurse Staffing and Quality of Patient Care
Periodic Health Evaluation, Value

Skin conditions
Heparin, Uses Treat Burn Injury

NOTE: BNP = B-Type natriuretic peptide; CYP450 = cytochrome P450; ICD = implantable cardioverter defibrillator; NT-proBNP = N-Terminal proBNP; SSRI = selective serotonin reuptake inhibitor.
SOURCE: AHRQ (2007e).

assessed in 2006. The committee then asked three additional health plans (Aetna, Kaiser Permanente, and WellPoint) and TEC, the ECRI Institute, and Hayes, Inc., if they had also conducted reviews of the 20 services that UnitedHealthcare had reviewed (Table 3-4). With only a few exceptions, each health plan and private firm had assessed the same 20 services that

BOX 3-3
Examples of Widely Adopted Health Interventions
Found to Be Ineffective or Harmful

- Antihistamines and oral decongestants to treat otitis media with effusion
- Autologous bone marrow transplant with high-dose chemotherapy for advanced breast cancer
- Chelation therapy to prevent or reverse atherosclerosis
- Diethylstilbestrol (DES) to prevent miscarriage
- Electronic fetal monitoring during labor without access to fetal scalp sampling
- Episiotomy (routine) for birth
- Extracranial-intracranial bypass to reduce the risk of ischemic stroke
- Fenfluramine plus phentermine to treat obesity
- Gastric bubble for morbid obesity
- Gastric freezing for peptic ulcer disease
- Home uterine activity monitoring to prevent preterm birth
- Hydralazine for chronic heart failure
- Lidocaine to prevent arrhythmia and sudden death in acute myocardial infarction
- Mammary artery ligation for coronary artery disease
- Optic nerve decompression surgery for nonarteritic anterior ischemic optic neuropathy
- Quinidine for suppressing recurrences of atrial fibrillation
- Radiation therapy for acne
- Spinal manipulation to treat migraine or cluster headaches
- Subcutaneous interferon alfa-2a to treat age-related macular degeneration
- Supplemental oxygen for healthy premature babies
- Thalidomide for sedation in pregnant women
- Traction to treat low back pain
- Triparanol (MER-29) for cholesterol reduction

NOTE: Adapted from Goodman (2004).
SOURCES: AHCPR (1990, 1993); BMJ (2004a,b,c); Coplen et al. (1990); Enkin et al. (1995); Feeny et al. (1986); Fletcher and Colditz (2002); Grimes (1993); The Ischemic Optic Neuropathy Decompression Trial Research Group (1995); Mello and Brennan (2001); Passamani (1991); Rossouw et al. (2002).

UnitedHealthcare had reviewed. All the services were recent health care innovations or new technologies. The committee was not able to determine if the duplicate independent reviews yielded similar results. Interestingly, AHRQ EPCs had reviewed only five of the topics.

TABLE 3-4 Duplicated Efforts by Selected Health Plans and Technology Assessment Firms, 2006

Type of Service	Health Plans				Technology Assessment Firms		
	United-Healthcare	Kaiser Permanente	Aetna	WellPoint	Hayes, Inc.	BCBSA TEC	ECRI
Screening							
Genetic testing to predict breast cancer recurrence	✓	✓	✓	✓	✓	✓	✓
Proteomic testing for ovarian cancer	✓		✓	✓	✓		✓
Virtual (computed tomography) colonoscopy	✓	✓	✓	✓	✓	✓	✓
Disease management							
Ambulatory blood pressure monitoring	✓	✓	✓	✓	✓	✓	✓
Intermittent intravenous insulin therapy	✓	✓		✓	✓		✓
Diagnosis							
CT angiography for suspected coronary artery disease	✓	✓	✓	✓	✓	✓	✓
Microvolt T-wave alternans	✓	✓	✓	✓	✓	✓	✓
Wireless capsule endoscopy	✓	✓	✓	✓	✓	✓	✓
Treatment							
Brachytherapy for various cancers: breast, ovarian, and prostate cancer and brain tumors	✓	✓	✓	✓	✓	✓	✓
Dysfunctional uterine bleeding and fibroids	✓	✓	✓	✓	✓	✓	✓
Fallopian tube occlusion for permanent contraception	✓	✓	✓	✓	✓		
Growth factor-mediated lumbar spinal fusion	✓	✓	✓	✓	✓		
Intracoronary brachytherapy	✓	✓	✓	✓	✓	✓	✓
Minimally invasive surgery for low back pain	✓	✓	✓	✓	✓	✓	✓
Photodynamic therapy for Barrett's esophagus and esophageal cancer	✓	✓	✓	✓	✓	✓	✓
Vagus nerve stimulation for intractable depression	✓	✓	✓	✓	✓	✓	✓

continued

TABLE 3-4 Continued

Type of Service	Health Plans United-Healthcare	Kaiser Permanente	Aetna	WellPoint	Technology Assessment Firms Hayes, Inc.	BCBSA TEC	ECRI
Devices							
Artificial total disc replacement for lumbar and cervical spine	✓	✓	✓	✓	✓		✓
Cochlear implants	✓	✓	✓	✓	✓	✓	✓
Total artificial heart	✓	✓	✓	✓	✓		✓
Total hip resurfacing arthroplasty	✓	✓	✓	✓	✓	✓	✓

NOTE: Not all reviews are comprehensive assessments. AHRQ EPCs have reviewed 5 of the 20 topics listed (ambulatory blood pressure monitoring, CT angiography, proteomic testing for ovarian cancer, spinal fusion for low back pain, and uterine fibroids). The Kaiser Permanente entries represent all Kaiser regions.

TABLE 3-5 Priority Setting Criteria That Selected Organizations Use

Organization	Cost	Disease Burden	Potential Impact	Public Interest or Controversy	New Evidence	Sufficient Evidence	Variation in Care
AHRQ[a]	✓	✓	✓	✓		✓	✓
BCBSA TEC[b]			✓	✓	✓		
CADTH	✓	✓	✓	✓		✓	
MedCAC and CMS			✓	✓	✓		
NICE	✓	✓	✓			✓	
NIH OMAR	✓	✓	✓	✓	✓	✓	
DERP[c]	✓						
USPSTF		✓	✓	✓	✓	✓	✓

NOTE: CADTH = Canadian Agency for Drugs and Technologies in Health; DERP = Drug Effectiveness Review Project; NICE = National Institute for Health and Clinical Excellence; NIH OMAR = National Institutes of Health Office of Medical Applications of Research.

[a]Also if relevant to federal health programs; specific plans to disseminate or otherwise use findings.

[b]Must be of interest to member plans.

[c]Also if multiple drugs are in the class, for off-label use, and for recent additions to drug class.

SOURCES: AHRQ (2007a,c,d); BCBSA (2007); CADTH (2005); CMS (2006); DERP (2007); Harris et al. (2001).

Methods Used to Identify High-Priority Topics

Selection Criteria

Many organizations report using the same general criteria to gauge the potential impact that an evidence assessment might have on clinical care and patient outcomes (Table 3-5) (Aronson, 2007; CADTH, 2005; Harris et al., 2001). These include the burden of disease (rates of disability, morbidity, or mortality), public controversy, cost (as related to the condition, as related to the procedure, or in the aggregate), potential impact, new evidence that might change previously held conclusions (new clinical trial results), the adequacy of the existing evidence, and unexplained variation in the use of services (Table 3-6). How these factors play into final priorities is not apparent.

One recent analysis found little congruence between the topics addressed by cost-effectiveness analyses, conducted from 1976 through 2001, and those conditions that caused the highest burden of disease or that were the top health concerns identified in the U.S. Surgeon General's report *Healthy People 2010* (HHS, 2000; Neumann et al., 2005). The effectiveness

TABLE 3-6 Definitions of Commonly Used Priority Setting Criteria

Criterion	Definition
Disease burden	Extent of disability, morbidity, or mortality imposed by a condition, including effects on patients, families, communities, and society overall
Controversy	Controversy or uncertainty around the topic and supporting data
Cost	Economic cost associated with the condition, procedure, treatment, or technology related to the number of people needing care, unit cost of care, or indirect costs
New evidence	New evidence with the potential to change conclusions from prior assessments
Potential impact	Potential to improve health outcomes (morbidity, mortality) and quality of life; improve decision making for patient or provider
Public or provider interest	Consumers, patients, clinicians, payers, and others want an assessment to inform decision making
Sufficient evidence	The available research literature provides adequate evidence to support an assessment
Variation in care	Potential to reduce unexplained variations in prevention, diagnosis, or treatment; the current use is outside the parameters of clinical evidence

reviews focused primarily on pharmaceuticals (40 percent) and surgical procedures (16 percent) and overrepresented cerebrovascular disease, diabetes, breast cancer, and HIV/AIDS, whereas they underrepresented depression and bipolar disorder, injuries, and substance abuse disorders. Similarly, a survey of European horizon-scanning agencies found little evidence that the organizations had operationalized all of their selection criteria (Douw and Vondeling, 2006).

FINDINGS

There is little solid basis at present for judging whether one method of selecting priorities is better than another. The Cochrane Collaboration and the USPSTF are currently reconsidering their approaches and may have insights to offer in the future (Cochrane Collaboration, 2007; Guirguis-Blake et al., 2007). Although AHRQ has handled a relatively small volume of nominations, it has considerable experience managing topic nominations for its effectiveness programs. The Program should learn from this experience.

New and emerging technologies are clearly high priorities for health plans. However, the Program should focus its priorities not only on what lies ahead, but also where there is meaningful potential to identify both new and established effective services. Several specific variables may be useful indicators of potential impacts, including burden of disease, cost, unexplained variations in use, and measures of disparities in health outcomes based on race and ethnicity.

The PSAC must consider how best to approach the setting of priorities for reviewing new and emerging technologies. There appear to be substantial efficiencies to be gained by reducing duplicative reviews of new technologies. Decision makers, especially in health plans and health systems, often need to decide quickly about whether to cover new and emerging technologies. Patients and providers want information on new health services as soon as they become available, often because manufacturers are pressing them to adopt a product or because patients have read direct-to-consumer advertising and want answers from their physicians. Yet, almost by definition, sufficient objective information about new and emerging technologies is seldom available. The PSAC should consider whether new and emerging technologies require the use of a different priority setting process—including the use of separate criteria—than other topics with more substantive evidence. There would be trade-offs in the resource and opportunity costs associated with two different processes.

There are few, if any, empirical data to suggest the optimal frequency for setting priorities or updating previous assessments. The Cochrane Collaboration recommends that systematic reviews be updated every two years and review groups send reminders and results of new literatures searches to prompt the authors (Higgins and Green, 2006). New knowledge, such as new evidence from recently conducted clinical trials, may trigger the need to reassess a previously considered topic, especially if it suggests the need for modifications to current clinical decision making. The PSAC should identify the quantitative and qualitative indicators that best signal the need for an update. Quantitative variables include, for example, significant changes in the magnitudes of effects (greater than 50 percent) for any primary or mortality outcome from the original systematic review (Shojania et al., 2007). Possible qualitative signals include new studies reporting substantial differences in effectiveness, new information about harm, or caveats about previously reported findings.

RECOMMENDATIONS

As noted earlier, the committee recommends that the Program appoint a PSAC to develop and implement a priority setting process that will identify those high-priority topics that merit systematic evidence assessment. This section draws from the research examined in this chapter, and based on the consensus of the committee, presents further recommendations for developing the Program's priority setting process. It also highlights key programmatic issues the PSAC must address including: PSAC membership, cultivating objectivity, scope, identifying potential topics, identifying priority topics, meeting frequency, and updating priorities and processes.

> **Recommendation: The Program should appoint a standing Priority Setting Advisory Committee (PSAC) to identify high-priority topics for systematic reviews of clinical effectiveness.**
>
> - The priority setting process should be open, transparent, efficient, and timely.
> - Priorities should reflect the potential for evidence-based practice to improve health outcomes across the life span, reduce the burden of disease and health disparities, and eliminate undesirable variations.
> - Priorities should also consider economic factors, such as the costs of treatment and the economic burden of disease.
> - The membership of the PSAC should include a broad mix of expertise and interests and be chosen to minimize committee bias due to conflicts of interest.

Guiding Principles

During the course of this study, the committee established a set of eight guiding principles for building the Program: accountability, consistency, efficiency, feasibility, objectivity, responsiveness, scientific rigor, and transparency. The principles are described in depth in Chapter 6. Five of the eight principles have particular salience for the Program's priority setting process and are described in Table 3-7.

Key Program Challenges

PSAC Membership

The PSAC would be an active body with ongoing responsibility for reviewing topic nominations, horizon scanning, and advising the Program on topics that merit priority systematic review. Members should be willing to make significant time commitments. There is limited research evidence to suggest the optimal composition or size of the PSAC. The committee believes that it should be sufficiently large to include all of the important stakeholders, but not too large so that it is unwieldy. The membership should mirror the Program's target audience, especially patients and consumers, clinicians, payers, and guideline developers, as well as individuals

TABLE 3-7 Principles for Setting Evidence Assessment Priorities

Principle	Implications for Priority Setting
Consistency—*methods are standardized and predictable*	The Program reliably uses standard processes and criteria.
Efficiency—*avoids waste and unnecessary duplication*	The process is simple.
Objectivity—*evidence based and without bias; conflict of interest is minimized*	The process is developed by a broadly representative group selected to ensure a balanced membership and minimal bias due to conflicts of interest.
Responsiveness—*addresses the information needs of decision makers*	The process cultivates input from key decision makers, particularly patients, clinicians, and guideline developers, and ensures up-to-date information. Evaluation of the process is a routine function.
Transparency—*methods are explicitly defined, consistently applied, and publicly available*	The process remains open, predictable, and explicitly defined, with fully documented standards and procedures.

with the appropriate expertise in the relevant content areas and technical methods. Maintaining expertise in all content areas will be impossible. The PSAC should consider using the CMS MedCAC approach. CMS sometimes recruits outside experts knowledgeable about a particular subject matter or methodologies to serve as nonvoting panelists to provide additional technical input to MedCAC deliberations (CMS MCAC Operations and Methodology Subcommittee, 2006).

The PSAC would require support staff to assist in efficient review of topic nominations. Staff expertise in library sciences and research databases will be especially important.

Cultivating Objectivity[2]

Objectivity implies balanced participation, oversight by a governance body, and standards that minimize conflicts of interest and other biases. The PSAC should not be dominated by special interests that can benefit materially or by intellectual biases that might favor one professional specialty over another (e.g., surgery versus medicine or ophthalmology versus optometry).

The use of transparent, well-documented, and standard procedures also contributes to perceptions of objectivity. Stakeholders are not likely to

---

[2]See Chapter 5, Developing Trusted Clinical Practice Guidelines, for further discussion of the factors involved in developing balance in an advisory group.

trust an unpredictable, opaque process. All deliberations should be open to encourage public participation and public confidence and to ensure the inclusion of a wide variety of perspectives. The PSAC should post key documents on its website, including meeting announcements and decisions concerning priorities, and should allow time for public comment on documents that support the priority setting process.

Scope

The PSAC should consider a broad range of topics, including, for example, new, emerging, and well-established health services across the full spectrum of health care (e.g., preventive interventions, diagnostic tests, treatments, rehabilitative therapies, and end-of-life care and palliation); community-based interventions such as immunization initiatives or programs to encourage smoking cessation; and research methods and data sources for the analysis of comparative effectiveness.

Identifying Potential Topics

There should be an open and inclusive topic nomination process that cultivates input from the key end users, such as the developers of guidelines and quality measures, patients, clinicians, and payers. Although the nomination process should not be overly burdensome to potential nominators, its methods, schedules, and information requirements should be standardized and predictable from year to year.

Topic nominations may not necessarily translate readily into answerable research questions. The AHRQ Effective Health Care Program requires nominators to provide standardized information in a template (Appendix C) that helps to clarify the focus of the suggested topic and to draw out the salient questions underlying the topic nomination. The PSAC should consider this approach.

Identifying Priority Topics

The PSAC should develop the selection criteria, with Program staff providing necessary research support. The committee believes that two considerations should be paramount in developing the selection criteria: (1) how well the topic reflects the clinical questions of patients and clinicians and (2) the potential for a large impact on clinical and other outcomes that matter the most to patients. It will be important to include criteria that indicate potential impacts, such as the burden of disease; economic factors, such as the costs of treatment and the economic burden of disease; unexplained variations; and measures of disparities in health outcomes based on race and ethnicity.

A strict, quantitative priority ranking may not be feasible given the range and complexity of potential topics regarding the management of specific health problems (e.g., back pain), specific patient populations (e.g., women under age 70 with advanced breast cancer who have undergone breast-conserving surgery), care settings (e.g., a specialized rehabilitation unit or a physician's office), the class of pharmacologic or nonpharmacologic treatment, the type of provider (e.g., a neurologist or a psychiatrist), and multiple patient outcomes (e.g., pain, return to work, and mortality).

Meeting Frequency

The PSAC should meet frequently enough so that its members may keep abreast of research discoveries, emerging technologies, and unexpected events that might affect the priorities that the PSAC establishes. There will be a continuing stream of new interventions and an ongoing imperative to determine if each new intervention is better than, comparable to, or worse than standard treatments. The priority setting process should be responsive to decision makers in a timely manner. It should also be routinely evaluated to ensure that it is fulfilling its purpose effectively and efficiently.

Updating Priorities and Processes

Research is iterative. New evidence can lead to new conclusions. The PSAC should develop a mechanism for revisiting past nominations, whether they have been rejected or accepted. On first consideration, the evidence for many topics will be insufficient to draw a conclusion on effectiveness.

REFERENCES

AHCPR (Agency for Health Care Policy and Research). 1990. *Extracranial-intracranial by-pass to reduce the risk of ischemic stroke: Health technology assessment report no. 6.* Rockville, MD: AHCPR.
———. 1993. *Intermittent positive pressure breathing: Old technologies rarely die.* Rockville, MD: AHCPR.
AHRQ (Agency for Healthcare Research and Quality). 2006. Solicitation for nominations for new primary and secondary health topics to be considered for review by the United States Preventive Services Task Force. *Federal Register* 71(15):3849-3850.
———. 2007a. *Effective health care home* http://effectivehealthcare.ahrq.gov/ (accessed August 7, 2007).
———. 2007b. Nominations of topics for Evidence-based Practice Centers. *Federal Register* 72(51):12618-12619.
———. 2007c. *Reports: Research reviews* http://effectivehealthcare.ahrq.gov/reports/reviews.cfm (accessed September 4, 2007).

———. 2007d. *Technology assessments* http://www.ahrq.gov/clinic/techix.htm (accessed September 4, 2007).

———. 2007e. *Topic index: A-Z Evidence-based Practice Centers (EPCs)* http://www.ahrq.gov/clinic/epcquick.htm (accessed September 4, 2007).

Aronson, N. 2007. *Approaches to priority setting: Identifying topics and selection (Submitted responses to the IOM HECS committee meeting, January 25, 2007).* Washington, DC.

BCBSA (Blue Cross and Blue Shield Association). 2007. *Blue Cross and Blue Shield Association's Technology Evaluation Center* http://www.bcbs.com/tec/index.html (accessed January 18, 2007).

BCBSA TEC (Blue Cross and Blue Shield Association Technology Evaluation Center). 2007. *2006 TEC Assessments (Volume 21)* http://www.bcbs.com/betterknowledge/tec/vols/#21 (accessed September 4, 2007).

BMJ. 2004a. Antihistamines and/or oral decongestants to treat otits media with effusion. *Clinical Evidence.* December. London, UK: BMJ Publishing Group.

———. 2004b. Fenfluramine plus phentermine to treat obesity. *Clinical Evidence.* December. London, UK: BMJ Publishing Group.

———. 2004c. Subcutaneous interferon alfa-2a to treat age-related macular degeneration. *Clinical Evidence* 88(12). December. London, UK: BMJ Publishing Group.

CADTH (Canadian Agency for Drugs and Technologies in Health). 2005. CADTH: HTA dictorate process documentation. In *CADTH: Topic identification, prioritization and refinement.* Ontario, Canada: CADTH.

CMS (Centers for Medicare & Medicaid Services). 2006. *Guidance for the public, industry, and CMS staff: Factors CMS considers in commissioning external technology assessments* http://www.cms.hhs.gov/mcd/ncpc_view_document.asp?id=7 (accessed January 18, 2007).

CMS MCAC Operations and Methodology Subcommittee (CMS Medicare Coverage Advisory Committee Operations and Methodology Subcommittee). 2006. *Process for evaluation of effectiveness and committee operations* http://www.cms.hhs.gov/FACA/Downloads/recommendations.pdf (accessed January 18, 2007).

Coates, V. 2007. *Stakeholders Forum (Presentation to the IOM HECS Committee Meeting, January 25, 2007).* Washington, DC.

Cochrane Collaboration. 2007. Setting priorities. *Cochrane News* (40), http://www.cochrane.org/newslett/CochraneNews_Aug07lowres.pdf (accessed September 12, 2007).

Coplen, S. E., E. M. Antman, J. A. Berlin, P. Hewitt, and T. C. Chalmers. 1990. Efficacy and safety of quinidine therapy for maintenance of sinus rhythm after cardioversion: A meta-analysis of randomized control trials. *Circulation* 82:1106-1116.

DERP (Drug Effectiveness Review Project). 2007. *Process* http://www.ohsu.edu/drugeffectiveness/process/index.htm (accessed September 4, 2007).

Douw, K., and H. Vondeling. 2006. Selection of new health technologies for assessment aimed at informing decision making: A survey among horizon scanning systems. *International Journal of Technology Assessment in Health Care* 22(2):177-183.

Enkin, M., M. Keirse, M. Renfrew, and J. Neilson. 1995. *A guide to effective care in pregnancy and childbirth.* 2nd ed. New York: Oxford University Press.

Feeny, D., G. Guyatt, and P. Tugwell eds. 1986. *Health care technology: Effectiveness, efficiency, and public policy.* Montreal, Canada: Institute for Research on Public Policy.

Fletcher, S. W., and G. A. Colditz. 2002. Failure of estrogen plus progestin therapy for prevention. *JAMA* 288:366-368.

Goodman, C. 2004. *HTA 101: Introduction to health technology assessment.* Falls Church, VA: The Lewin Group.

Grimes, D. A. 1993. Technology follies: The uncritical acceptance of medical innovation. *JAMA* 269(23):3030-3033.

Guirguis-Blake, J., N. Calonge, T. Miller, A. Siu, S. Teutsch, and E. Whitlock. 2007. Current processes of the U.S. Preventive Services Task Force: Refining evidence-based recommendation development. *Annals of Internal Medicine* 147(2).

Harris, R. P., M. Helfand, S. H. Woolf, K. N. Lohr, C. D. Mulrow, S. M. Teutsch, and D. Atkins. 2001. Current methods of the U.S. Preventive Services Task Force: A review of the process. *American Journal of Preventive Medicine* 20(3 Suppl):21-35.

HHS (U.S. Department of Health and Human Services). 2000. *Healthy people 2010: Understanding and improving health.* 2nd ed. Washington, DC: U.S. Government Printing Office.

Higgins, J. T., and S. Green. 2006. *Cochrane handbook for systematic reviews of interventions 4.2.6 [updated September 2006],* The Cochrane Library, Issue 4, 2006. Chichester, UK: John Wiley & Sons, Ltd.

IOM (Institute of Medicine). 1990. *National priorities for the assessment of clinical conditions and medical technologies: Report of a pilot study.* Edited by Lara, M. E., and C. Goodman. Washington, DC: National Academy Press.

———. 1992. *Setting priorities for health technologies assessment: A model process.* Edited by Donaldson, M. S., and H. C. Sox. Washington, DC: National Academy Press.

———. 1995. *Setting priorities for clinical practice guidelines.* Edited by Field, M. J. Washington, DC: National Academy Press.

———. 2003. *Priority areas for national action: Transforming health care quality.* Edited by Adams, K., and J. M. Corrigan. Washington, DC: The National Academies Press.

The Ischemic Optic Neuropathy Decompression Trial Research Group. 1995. Optic nerve decompression surgery for nonarteritic anterior ischemic optic neuropathy (NAION) is not effective and may be harmful. *JAMA* 273(8):625-632.

Mello, M. M., and T. A. Brennan. 2001. The controversy over high-dose chemotherapy with autologous bone marrow transplant for breast cancer. *Health Affairs* 20(5):101-117.

Murphy, K., C. Packer, A. Stevens, and S. Simpson. 2007. Effective early warning systems for new and emerging health technologies: Developing an evaluation framework and an assessment of current systems. *International Journal of Technology Assessment in Health Care* 23(3):324-330.

NIH Consensus Development Program (National Institutes of Health Consensus Development Program). 2005. *About the National Institutes of Health (NIH) Consensus Development Program (CDP)* http://consensus.nih.gov/ABOUTCDP.htm#topic (accessed January 18, 2007).

———. 2007. *Previous conference statements* http://consensus.nih.gov/PREVIOUSSTATEMENTS. htm (accessed September 4, 2007).

Neumann, P. J., A. B. Rosen, D. Greenberg, N. V. Olchanski, R. Pande, R. H. Chapman, P. W. Stone, J. Ondategui-Parra, J. Nadai, J. E. Siegel, and M. C. Weinstein. 2005. Can we better prioritize resources for cost-utility research? *Medical Decision Making* 25(4):429-436.

Noorani, H. Z., D. R. Husereau, R. Boudreau, and B. Skidmore. 2007. Priority setting for health technology assessments: A systematic review of current practical approaches. *International Journal of Technology Assessment in Health Care* 23(3):310-315.

OTA (U.S. Congress Office of Technology Assessment). 1994. *Identifying health technologies that work: Searching for evidence.* Washington, DC: Government Printing Office.

Oxman, A. D., H. J. Schünemann, and A. Fretheim. 2006. Improving the use of research evidence in guideline development: 2. Priority setting. *Health Research Policy and Systems* 4(14).

Passamani, E. 1991. Clinical trials: Are they ethical? *New England Journal of Medicine* 324(22):1589-1592.

Phelps, C., and S. Parente. 1990. Priority setting in medical technology and medical practice assessment. *Medical Care* 28:703-723.

Rettig, R., P. Jacobsen, C. Farquhar, and W. Aubrey. 2007. *False hope: Bone marrow transplantation for breast cancer.* New York: Oxford University Press.

Rossouw, J. E., G. L. Anderson, and R. L. Prentice. 2002. Risks and benefits of estrogen plus progestin in healthy postmenopausal women: Principal results from the Women's Health Initiative randomized controlled trial. *JAMA* 288:321-333.

Sassi, F. 2003. Setting priorities for the evaluation of health interventions: When theory does not meet practice. *Health Policy (Amsterdam, Netherlands)* 63(2):141-154.

Shojania, K. G., M. Sampson, M. T. Ansari, J. Ji, S. Doucette, and D. Moher. 2007. How quickly do systematic reviews go out of date? A survival analysis. *Annals of Internal Medicine* 147:224-233.

4

Systematic Reviews: The Central Link Between Evidence and Clinical Decision Making

If, as is sometimes supposed, science consisted in nothing but the laborious accumulation of facts, it would soon come to a standstill, crushed, as it were, under its own weight. Two processes are thus at work side by side, the reception of new material and the digestion and assimilation of the old. . . . The work which deserves, but I am afraid does not always receive, the most credit is that in which discovery and explanation go hand in hand, in which not only are new facts presented, but their relation to old ones is pointed out.

J. W. Strutt Lord Rayleigh
Address to the British Association for the Advancement of Science
(Rayleigh, 1884, p. 1)

More than a decade has passed since it was first shown that patients have been harmed by failure to prepare scientifically defensible reviews of existing research evidence. There are now many examples of the dangers of this continuing scientific sloppiness. Organizations and individuals concerned about improving the effectiveness and safety of health care now look to systematic reviews of research—not individual studies—to inform their judgments.

Iain Chalmers
Academia's Failure to Support Systematic Reviews
(Chalmers, 2005)

Abstract: This chapter provides the committee's findings and recommendations for conducting systematic evidence reviews under the aegis of a proposed national clinical effectiveness assessment program ("the Program"). The chapter reviews the origins of systematic review methods and describes the fundamental components of systematic reviews and the shortcomings of current efforts. Under the status quo, the quality of the reviews is variable, methods are poorly documented, and findings are often unreliable. The committee recommends that the Program establish evidence-based, methodological standards for systematic reviews, including standard terminology for characterizing the strength of evidence and a standard reporting format for systematic reviews. Once Program stan-

dards are established, the Program should fund only those reviewers who commit to and consistently meet the standards. The committee found that the new science of systematic reviews has made great strides, but more methodological research is needed. Investing in the science of research synthesis will increase the quality and the value of the evidence provided in systematic reviews. It is not clear whether there are sufficient numbers of qualified researchers to conduct high-quality reviews. The capacity of the workforce should be assessed and expanded, if needed.

Systematic reviews are central to scientific inquiry into what is known and not known about what works in health care (Glasziou and Haynes, 2005; Helfand, 2005; Mulrow and Lohr, 2001; Steinberg and Luce, 2005). In 1884, J. W. Strutt Lord Rayleigh, who later won a Nobel prize in physics, observed that the synthesis and explanation of past discoveries are integral to future progress (Rayleigh, 1884). Yet, more than a century later, Antman and colleagues (1992) and Lau and colleagues (1992) clearly demonstrated that this message was still largely ignored, with the potential for great harm to patients. In a series of meta-analyses examining the treatment of myocardial infarction, the researchers concluded that clinicians need better access to syntheses of the results of existing studies to formulate clinical recommendations. Today, systematic reviews of the available evidence remain an often undervalued scientific discipline.

This chapter has three principal objectives: (1) to describe the fundamental components of a systematic review, (2) to present the committee's recommendations for conducting systematic evidence reviews under the aegis of a proposed national clinical effectiveness assessment program ("the Program"), and (3) to highlight the key challenges in producing high-quality systematic reviews.

BACKGROUND

What Is a Systematic Review?

A systematic review is a scientific investigation that focuses on a specific question and uses explicit, preplanned scientific methods to identify, select, assess, and summarize similar but separate studies (Haynes et al., 2006; West et al., 2002). It may or may not include a quantitative synthesis of the results from separate studies (meta-analysis). A meta-analysis quantitatively combines the results of similar studies in an attempt to allow inference from the sample of studies included to the population of interest. This report uses the term "systematic review" to describe reviews that incorporate meta-analyses as well as reviews that present the study data descriptively rather than inferentially.

Individual studies rarely provide definitive answers to clinical effectiveness questions (Cook et al., 1997). If it is conducted properly, a systematic review should make obvious the gap between what is known about the effectiveness of a particular service and what clinicians and patients want to know (Helfand, 2005). As such, systematic reviews are also critical to the development of an agenda for further primary research because they reveal where the evidence is insufficient and new information is needed (Neumann, 2006). Without systematic reviews, researchers may miss promising leads or pursue questions that have already been answered (Mulrow et al., 1997). In addition, systematic reviews provide an essential bridge between the body of research evidence and the development of clinical guidance.

Key U.S. Producers and Users of Systematic Reviews

This section briefly describes the variety of contexts in which key U.S. organizations produce or use systematic reviews (Table 4-1). The ultimate purposes of systematic reviews vary and include health coverage decisions, practice guidelines, regulatory approval of new pharmaceuticals or medical devices, clinical research or program planning. Within the federal government, the users include the Agency for Healthcare Research and Quality (AHRQ), the Centers for Medicare & Medicaid Services (CMS), the Medicare Evidence Development and Coverage Advisory Committee (MedCAC), the Centers for Disease Control and Prevention (CDC), the U.S. Food and Drug Administration (FDA), the Substance Abuse and Mental Health Administration (SAMHSA), the U.S. Preventive Services Task Force (USPSTF), and the Veterans Health Administration (VHA).

AHRQ plays a lead role in producing systematic reviews through its program of Evidence-based Practice Centers (EPCs) as a part of its Effective Health Care Program. EPCs produce systematic reviews for professional medical societies and several federal agencies, including CMS and the National Institutes of Health (NIH) Consensus Development Conferences, as well as a variety of other public and private requestors, such as the USPSTF and the American Heart Association. The reviews cover a broad range of topics, including the effectiveness and safety of health care interventions, emergency preparedness, research methods, and approaches to improving the quality and delivery of health care.[1] The AHRQ Effective Health Care Program produces comparative effectiveness studies on surgical procedures, medical devices, and medical therapies in 10 priority areas (Slutsky, 2007).

The CDC conducts or sponsors systematic effectiveness reviews to evaluate and make recommendations on population-based and public

---

[1] See Table 3-3 in Chapter 3 for a list of recent EPC studies.

TABLE 4-1 Key U.S. Producers and Users of Systematic Reviews

	Government Agencies						
Component	AHRQ	USPSTF	SAMHSA	FDA	VHA	CMS MedCAC	CDC
Activity							
• Produces reviews	✓				✓		✓
• Sponsors or purchases reviews	✓	✓			✓	✓	✓
Principal use							
• Development of practice guidelines and recommendations	✓	✓	✓		✓		✓
• Decisions regarding health coverage	✓	✓			✓	✓	
• Regulatory approval				✓			

NOTE: BCBSA TEC = Blue Cross and Blue Shield Association Technology Evaluation Center.

health interventions and to improve the underlying research methods (CDC, 2007).

The Blue Cross and Blue Shield Association (BCBSA) Technology Evaluation Center (TEC) produces systematic reviews that assess medical technologies for decision makers in its member plans but also provides the results of these reviews to the public for free.[2] Many other health plans look to private research organizations, such as the ECRI Institute and Hayes, Inc., that produce systematic evidence assessments available by subscription or for purchase (ECRI, 2006a,b; Hayes, Inc., 2007). Because the reviews are proprietary, they are not free to the public and the subscription fees are considerable. At Hayes, Inc., for example, subscriptions range from $10,000 to $300,000, depending on the size of the subscribing organizations and the types of products licensed.[3]

The Cochrane Collaboration is an international effort that produces systematic reviews of health interventions; 11 percent (nearly 1,700 individuals) of its active contributors are in the United States (Allen and Clarke, 2007). Cochrane reviews are available by subscription to *The Cochrane Library*, and abstracts are available for free through PubMed or www.cochrane.org.

---

[2]See http://www.bcbs.com/betterknowledge/tec/.
[3]Personal communication, W. S. Hayes, Hayes, Inc., August 29, 2007.

| Private Research Firms | | | Other Entities | | | |
ECRI Institute	BCBSA TEC	Hayes, Inc.	Cochrane Collaboration	Health Plans	Specialty Societies	Manufacturers
✓	✓	✓	✓	✓	✓	✓
				✓	✓	✓
✓	✓	✓	✓		✓	✓
✓	✓	✓	✓	✓		✓
						✓

Professional medical societies often sponsor or conduct evidence reviews as the first step in developing a practice guideline. These include, for example, the American College of Physicians, several cardiology groups (the American College of Cardiology, the American College of Chest Physicians, and the American Heart Association), the American Academy of Neurology, and the American Society of Clinical Oncology.

Origins of Systematic Review Methods

The term "meta-analysis" was first used by social scientists in the 1970s to describe the process of identifying a representative set of studies of a given topic and summarizing their results quantitatively. In a groundbreaking 1976 assessment of treatment for depression, Glass (1976) first used the term "meta-analysis" to describe what is now referred to as systematic review. Textbooks describing the concept and methods of systematic reviews (Cooper and Rosenthal, 1980; Glass et al., 1981; Hedges and Olkin, 1985; Light and Pillemer, 1984; Rosenthal, 1978; Sutton et al., 2000), and research articles exploring issues such as publication bias followed during that and the subsequent decade.

Subsequently, as quantitative syntheses started to include qualitative summaries and medical scientists adopted the methods, a new terminology emerged. Richard Peto and colleagues used the term "overview" for the new combined approach (Early Breast Cancer Trialists' Collaborative Group, 1988). Chalmers and Altman (1995) appear to have introduced the term "systematic review" in their book *Systematic Reviews*. They also suggested that the term "meta-analysis" be restricted to the statistical summary of the results of studies identified as a product of the review process (Chalmers and Altman, 1995). Confusion over terminology persists today, perhaps because the methods grew up in the social sciences and only later were embraced by the medical sciences.

The statistical methods underlying the quantitative aspects of systematic review—i.e., meta-analysis—date to the early 20th century, when statisticians started developing methods for combining the findings from separate but similar studies. In 1904, using new statistical methods, Karl Pearson (1904) combined research on the impact of inoculation against enteric fever on mortality in five communities. In a 1907 study on the prevalence of typhoid, Goldberger (1907) again used quantitative synthesis.

Social scientists were the first to use methods to critically synthesize results to allow statistical inference from a sample a population. As early as 1940, Pratt and colleagues (1940) at Duke University published a critical synthesis of more than 60 years of research on extrasensory perception.

Systematic reviews in the health care arena were comparatively slow to catch on, and the growth in their development and use coincided with the general rise of evidence-based medicine (Guyatt, 1991). The early implementers of systematic reviews were those who conducted clinical trials and who saw the need to summarize data from multiple effectiveness trials, many of them with very small sample sizes (Yusuf et al., 1985). In the 1970s, Iain Chalmers organized the first major collaborative effort to develop a clinical trials evidence base, beginning with the Oxford Database of Perinatal Trials (Chalmers et al., 1986). This subsequently led to two major compilations of systematic reviews of clinical trials, one of pregnancy and childbirth (Chalmers et al., 1989) and one of the newborn period (Sinclair and Bracken, 1992). The growth of bioinformatics, specifically, electronic communication, data storage, and improved indexing and retrieval of publications, allowed this collaborative effort in the perinatal field to expand further. In 1993, the Cochrane Collaboration was formed (Dickersin and Manheimer, 1998) with the aim of synthesizing information from studies of interventions on all health topics.

Up to this time, literature reviews were often used to assess the effectiveness of health care interventions, but empiric research also began to reveal problems in their execution. The methods underlying the reviews were often neither objective nor transparent (Mulrow, 1987; Oxman and Guyatt, 1988); and they did not routinely use scientific methods to identify, assess, and synthesize information. The approach to deciding which literature should be included and which findings should be presented was subjective and nonsystematic. The reviews may have provided thoughtful, readable discussions of a topic, but the conclusions were generally not credible.

The following sections of the chapter describe the fundamentals of conducting a scientifically rigorous systematic review and then provide the committee's findings on current efforts.

FUNDAMENTALS OF A SYSTEMATIC REVIEW

Although researchers use a variety of terms to describe the building blocks of a systematic review, the fundamentals are well established (AHRQ EPC Program, 2007; Counsell, 1997; EPC Coordinating Center, 2005; Haynes et al., 2006; Higgins and Green, 2006; Khan and Kleijnen, 2001; Khan et al., 2001a,b; West et al., 2002).[4] Five basic steps (listed below) should be followed, and the key decisions that comprise each step of the review should be clearly documented.

Step 1: Formulate the research question.
Step 2: Construct an analytic (or logic) framework.
Step 3: Conduct a comprehensive search for evidence.
Step 4: Critically appraise the evidence.
Step 5: Synthesize the body of evidence.

The following sections briefly describe each of these steps in the process.

Step 1: Formulate the Research Question

The foundation of a good systematic review is a well-formulated, clearly defined, answerable question. As such, it guides the analytic (or logic) framework for the review, the overall research protocol (i.e., the search for relevant evidence, decisions about which types of evidence should be used, and how best to identify the evidence), and the critical appraisal of the relevant evidence. The objective, in this first step, is to define a precise, unambiguous answerable research question.

Richardson and colleagues (1995) coined the mnemonic PICO (population, intervention, comparison, and outcome of interest) to help ensure that explicit attention is paid to the four key elements of an evidence question.[5,6]

---

[4]Unless otherwise noted, this section draws from these references.

[5]Personal communication, W. S. Richardson, Boonshoft School of Medicine, Wright State University, October 3, 2007.

[6]A recent draft version of an AHRQ comparative effectiveness methods manual proposes expanding the PICO format to PICOTS, adding "t" for timing and "s" for settings (AHRQ, 2007a).

Table 4-2 shows examples of how the PICO format can guide the building of a research question.

The characteristics of the study population, such as age, sex, severity of illness, and presence of comorbidities, usually vary among studies and can be important factors in the effect of an intervention. Health care interventions may have numerous outcomes of interest. The research question should be formulated so that it addresses all outcomes—beneficial and adverse—that matter to patients, clinicians, payers, developers of practice guidelines, and others who may be affected (Schünemann et al., 2006). For example, treatments for prostate cancer may affect mortality; but patients are also interested in learning about potential harmful treatment effects, such as urinary incontinence and impotence. Imaging tests for Alzheimer's disease may lead to the early diagnosis of the condition, but patients and the patients' caregivers may be particularly interested in whether an early diagnosis improves cognitive outcomes or quality of life.

Many researchers suggest that decision makers be directly involved in formulating the question to ensure that the systematic review is relevant and can inform decision making (Lavis et al., 2005; Schünemann et al., 2006). The questions posed by end users must sometimes be reframed to be answerable by clinical research studies.

TABLE 4-2 PICO Format for Formulating an Evidence Question

PICO Component	Tips for Building Question	Example
Patient population or problem	"How would I describe this group of patients?" • *Balance precision with brevity*	"In patients with heart failure from dilated cardiomyopathy who are in sinus rhythm . . ."
Intervention (a cause, prognostic factor, treatment, etc.)	"Which main intervention is of interest?" • *Be specific*	". . . would adding anticoagulation with warfarin to standard heart failure therapy . . ."
Comparison intervention (if necessary)	"What is the main alternative to be compared with the intervention?" • *Be specific*	". . . when compared with standard therapy alone . . ."
Outcomes	"What do I hope the intervention will accomplish?" "What could this exposure really affect?" • *Be specific*	". . . lead to lower mortality or morbidity from thromboembolism? Is this enough to be worth the increased risk of bleeding?"

SOURCE: Adapted from the *Evidence-based Practice Center Partner's Guide* (EPC Coordinating Center, 2005).

Step 2: Construct an Analytic Framework

Once the research question is established, it should be articulated in an analytic framework that clearly lays out the chain of logic underlying the case for the health intervention of interest. The complexity of the analysis will vary depending on the number of linkages between the intervention and the outcomes of interest. For preventive services, there may be multiple steps between, for example, screening for a disease and reductions in morbidity and mortality. Figure 4-1 shows the generic analytic framework

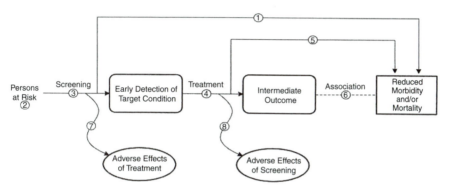

FIGURE 4-1 Analytic framework used by the U.S. Preventive Services Task Force. NOTE: Generic analytic framework for screening topics. Numbers refer to key questions as follow: (1) Is there direct evidence that screening reduces morbidity and/or mortality? (2) What is the prevalence of disease in the target groups? Can a high-risk group be reliably identified? (3) Can the screening test accurately detect the target condition? (a) What are the sensitivity and specificity of the test? (b) Is there significant variation between examiners in how the test is performed? (c) In actual screening programs, how much earlier are patients identified and treated? (4) Does treatment reduce the incidence of the intermediate outcome? (a) Does treatment work under ideal, clinical trial conditions? (b) How do the efficacy and effectiveness of treatments compare in community settings? (5) Does treatment improve health outcomes for people diagnosed clinically? (a) How similar are people diagnosed clinically to those diagnosed by screening? (b) Are there reasons to expect people diagnosed by screening to have even better health outcomes than those diagnosed clinically? (6) Is there intermediate outcome reliability associated with reduced morbidity and/or mortality? (7) Does screening result in adverse effects? (a) Is the test acceptable to patients? (b) What are the potential harms, and how often do they occur? (8) Does treatment result in adverse effects?
SOURCE: Reprinted from the *American Journal of Preventive Medicine*, 20(3) Harris, R. P., M. Helfand, S. H. Woolf, K. N. Lohr, C. D. Mulrow, S. M. Teutsch, and D. Atkins, Current methods of the US Preventive Services Task Force: A review of the process, 21-35, Copyright 2007, with permission from Elsevier.

that the USPSTF uses to assess screening interventions. It makes explicit the population at risk (left side of the figure), preventive services, diagnostic or therapeutic interventions, and intermediate and health outcomes to be considered (Harris et al., 2001). It also illustrates the chain of logic that the evidence must support to link the service to potential health outcomes: the arrows (linkages), labeled with a service or treatment, represent the questions that the evidence must answer; dotted lines represent associations; and rectangles represent the intermediate outcomes (rounded corners) or the health states (square corners) by which those linkages are measured.

The overarching linkage (Arrow 1) above the primary framework represents evidence that directly links screening to changes in health outcomes. For example, a randomized controlled trial (RCT) of screening for Chlamydia established a direct, causal connection between screening and reductions in the incidence of pelvic inflammatory disease (Meyers et al., 2007; Scholes et al., 1996). That is, a single body of evidence established the connection between the preventive service (screening) and the health outcome (reduced morbidity).

When direct evidence is lacking or is of insufficient quality to be convincing, the USPSTF relies on a chain of linkages to assess the likely effectiveness of a service. These linkages correspond to key questions about the screening test accuracy (Arrow 3), the efficacy of treatment (Arrows 4 and 5 for intermediate and health outcomes, respectively), and the association between intermediate measures and health outcomes (Dotted Line 6). A similar analytic framework can be constructed for questions of drug treatment, devices, behavior change, procedures, health care delivery, or any type of health intervention used in a population or in individuals.

Deciding Which Evidence to Use: Study Selection Criteria

What constitutes evidence that a health care service is highly effective? As noted in Chapter 1, scientists view evidence as knowledge that is explicit, systematic, and replicable. However, patients, clinicians, payers, and other decision makers have different perspectives on what constitutes evidence of effectiveness. For example, some may view the scientific evidence as demonstrating what works under ideal circumstances but not necessarily under a particular set of real world circumstances. A variety of factors can affect the applicability of a particular RCT to individual clinical decisions or circumstances, including patient factors, such as comorbidities, underlying risk, adherence to therapies, disease stage and severity, health insurance coverage, and demographics; intervention factors, such as care setting, level of training, timing and quality of the intervention, and an array of other factors (Atkins, 2007).

The choice of study designs to be included in a systematic review should be based on the type of research question being asked and should have the goal of minimizing bias (Glasziou et al., 2004; Oxman et al., 2006). Table 4-3 provides examples of research questions and the types of evidence that are the most appropriate for addressing them. RCTs can answer questions about the efficacy of screening, preventive, and therapeutic interventions. Although RCTs can best answer questions about the potential harms from interventions, observational study designs, such as cohort studies, case series, or case control studies, may be all that are available or possible for the evaluation of rare or long-term outcomes.[7] In fact, because harms from interventions are often rare or occur far in the future, a systematic review of observational research may be the best approach to identifying reliable evidence on potential rare harms (or benefits).

Observational studies are generally the most appropriate for answering questions related to prognosis, diagnostic accuracy, incidence, prevalence, and etiology (Chou and Helfand, 2005; Tatsioni et al., 2005). Cohort studies and case series are useful for examining long-term outcomes because RCTs may not monitor patients beyond the primary outcome of interest or for rare outcomes because they generally have small numbers of participants. Case series are often used, for example, to identify the potential long-term harms of new types of radiotherapy. Similarly, the best evidence on potential harms related to oral contraceptive use (e.g., an increased risk of thromboembolism) may be from nonrandomized cohort studies or case-control studies (Glasziou et al., 2004).

Many systematic reviews use a best evidence approach that allows the use of broader inclusion criteria when higher-quality evidence is lacking (Atkins et al., 2005). In these cases, the systematic reviews consider observational studies because, at a minimum, noting the available evidence helps to delineate what is known and what is not known about the effectiveness of the intervention in question. By highlighting the gaps in knowledge, the review establishes the need for better quality evidence and helps to prioritize research topics.

For intervention effectiveness questions for which RCTs form the highest level of evidence, it is essential to fully document the rationale for including nonrandomized evidence in a review. Current practice does not meet this standard, however. Researchers have found, for example, that 30 of 49 EPC reports that included observational studies did not disclose the rationale for doing so (Norris and Atkins, 2005).

---

[7]See Chapter 1 for the definitions of the types of experimental and observational studies.

TABLE 4-3 Matching the Clinical Question with the Appropriate Evidence

Type of Question	Example of Question	Type of Evidence[a]
Screening or early diagnosis	Is prostate-specific antigen screening for the detection of prostate cancer in low-risk populations effective in reducing mortality?	RCTs
	Does early diagnosis by use of a PET[b] scan result in improved cognitive ability for patients with Alzheimer's disease?	RCTs
Etiology	Does smoking cause lung cancer?	Cohort studies, case-control studies
Diagnostic accuracy	Does a PET scan diagnose Alzheimer's disease more accurately than a standard clinical evaluation?	Case series (RCTs desirable but unlikely)
Prognosis	What is the likelihood for fertility loss in a premenopausal woman receiving chemotherapy for breast cancer?	RCTs, cohort studies
	How long do patients remain insulin independent after pancreatic islet cell transplantation for Type I diabetes mellitus?	Cohort studies, case series
Preventive or therapeutic effectiveness[c]	Is bevacizumab (Avastin) as effective as ranibizumab (Lucentis) in delaying the progression of acute macular degeneration?	RCTs
	How does surgical implantation of an artificial lumbar disc compare with lumbar spinal fusion for pain reduction in patients with degenerative disc disease?	RCTs
	Is external beam radiation more effective than watchful waiting in reducing mortality from prostate cancer?	RCTs
Safety or potential harm	What proportion of postmenopausal women receiving calcium and vitamin D supplements develop kidney stones?	RCTs, cohort studies, case-control studies
	Is robotic-assisted radical prostatectomy more likely to lead to urinary incontinence than laparoscopicic-assisted radical prostatectomy?	RCTs, cohort studies, case-control studies

[a]Systematic reviews of the "best" evidence are more reliable than evidence from a single study, regardless of the clinical question being asked.

[b]PET = positron emission tomography.

[c]Includes drugs, devices, procedures, physical therapy, counseling, behavior change, and systems change in head-to-head comparisons and comparisons with standard interventions, placebo or sham treatments, or no intervention.

SOURCE: Adapted from the work of Dickersin (2007).

Dearth of Evidence

For surgical procedures, population-based public health measures, quality improvement strategies, and many other health care interventions, relevant, randomized evidence is frequently unavailable (Norris and Atkins, 2005).

Indeed, the evidence base on the effectiveness of most health services is sparse (BCBSA, 2007; Congressional Budget Office, 2007; The Health Industry Forum, 2006; IOM, 2007; Medicare Payment Advisory Commission, 2007; Wilensky, 2006). Well-designed, well-conducted studies of the effectiveness of most health care services are the exception, and the available research evidence falls far short of answering many questions that are important to patients and providers (Tunis, 2006). Although the FDA reviews prescription drugs for their short-term safety and efficacy, medical devices, surgical procedures and implants, diagnostic tests, common off-label uses of pharmaceuticals, and new combinations of approved uses of pharmaceuticals do not receive comparable reviews. Moreover, the FDA reviews do not consider evidence on whether the benefits of using a drug or a device outweigh the potential harms in individual patients or population groups. Effectiveness data for major subpopulations, including children, elderly people, African Americans, and Hispanics, are rarely available.

Commonly, researchers carefully review hundreds of references from the literature, only to conclude that no eligible study that directly addresses the question of interest exists. For example, in a review of the evidence on how best to determine if acute conjunctivitis is viral or bacterial in origin, the investigators were unable to identify evidence of the diagnostic validity of clinical signs, symptoms, or both in distinguishing bacterial conjunctivitis from viral conjunctivitis (Rietveld et al., 2003).

Neumann and colleagues (2005) reviewed the availability and quality of evidence for 69 medical devices, surgical procedures, and other medical therapies that were subject to national Medicare coverage determinations from 1998 to 2003.[8] The researchers found good evidence on health outcomes for only 11 of the 69 technologies (16 percent) (Table 4-4). For more than 29 technologies, there was either no evidence at all (6 technologies) or poor-quality evidence (23 technologies) because of a limited number of studies, the weak power of the studies, flaws in the design or the conduct of the studies, or missing information on important health outcomes. The evidence was considered "fair" for 29 technologies (42 percent). See Box 4-1 for a list of the technologies with poor or no evidence.

The Medicare experience closely mirrors that at the USPSTF. The

---

[8]Excluding 13 coverage decisions that were omitted because they involved minor coding or language changes ($n = 7$), exceptional circumstances ($n = 3$), or incomplete Centers for Medicare & Medicaid Services decision memoranda ($n = 3$).

TABLE 4-4 Quality of Evidence for Technologies Subject to Medicare National Coverage Determinations, 1998-2003

Rating	Number of Technologies	Percent
All technologies	69	100
Good	11	16
Fair	29	42
Poor	23	33
Unavailable	6	9

NOTE: The ratings are based on USPSTF criteria. "Good" indicates consistent results from well-designed, well-conducted studies with representative populations. "Fair" indicates sufficient evidence to determine effect on health outcomes but the evidence is limited by the number, quality, or consistency of the individual studies. "Poor" indicates insufficient evidence on effects on health outcomes because of a limited number of studies or the weak power of the studies, flaws in study design or conduct, or lack of information on important health outcomes.
SOURCE: Neumann et al. (2007).

USPSTF currently has 114 recommendations on the use of clinical preventive services by specific population groups (e.g., men ages 50 to 70 years or women older than age 65 years). For almost 40 percent (44 of 114) of the recommendations, the USPSTF concluded that the evidence was insufficient to determine if the service had an effect on health outcomes for the specified population because of a limited number of studies or the weak power of the studies, important flaws in the design or conduct of the studies, gaps in the chain of evidence, or a lack of information on important health outcomes (Barton, 2007; USPSTF, 2007). Box 4-2 lists prevention topics with insufficient evidence for one or more population subgroups. These include, for example, routine use of testing for human papillomavirus as a primary screening test for cervical cancer; screening of asymptomatic individuals for lung cancer by the use of low-dose computerized tomography, chest X-ray, sputum cytology, or a combination of these tests; and routine screening for prostate cancer by prostate-specific antigen testing or digital rectal examination.

New Sources of Evidence

There is growing interest in using sources of evidence such as large clinical and administrative databases based on electronic health records, registries, and other sources (AHRQ, 2007b; Perlin and Kupersmith, 2007). As health information technology advances, these sources of evidence will grow richer and the information contained in them should be mined as appropriate. Large data sets are especially useful for examining questions of incidence, prognosis, diagnosis, harms, related risks, effects of complex

---

BOX 4-1
Medicare National Coverage Decisions with Poor Evidence

- Air-fluidized beds for pressure ulcers
- Autologous stem cell transplantation for AL amyloidosis
- Biofeedback for urinary incontinence
- Cardiac pacemakers
- Cryosurgical salvage therapy for recurrent prostate cancer
- Electrical bioimpedence for cardiac output monitoring
- Electrical stimulation for fracture healing
- Electrodiagnostic sensory nerve conduction threshold
- Home biofeedback for urinary incontinence
- Liver transplantation for malignancies other than hepatocellular carcinoma
- Noninvasive positive-pressure respiratory-assist devices for chronic obstructive pulmonary disease
- Ocular photodynamic therapy with verteporfin for macular degeneration
- Pneumatic compression pumps for venous insufficiency
- Positron emission tomography fluorodeoxyglucose (FDG) for Alzheimer's disease/dementia
- Positron emission tomography (FDG) for breast cancer
- Positron emission tomography (FDG) for soft tissue sarcoma
- Positron emission tomography scanner technology
- Prolotherapy for chronic low back pain
- Transmyocardial revascularization for severe angina
- Warm-Up Wound Therapy (noncontact normothermic wound therapy)

NOTE: Evidence was considered "poor" if it was insufficient to assess the effects on health outcomes because of the limited number of studies or weak power of the studies, flaws in study design or conduct, or lack of information on important health outcomes.
SOURCE: Neumann et al. (2007).

---

patterns of comorbidities, and the effects of genetic variation (Francis and Perlin, 2006; IOM, 2007; Stewart et al., 2007). Mathematical modeling, Bayesian statistics, and decision modeling have also been heralded as having great future potential in better understanding health care effectiveness and risks (Claxton et al., 2005; Eddy, 2007). These types of evidence will pose significant challenges, but are likely to prove essential to understanding and improving health and health care systems.

Step 3: Conduct a Comprehensive Search for Evidence

The search for the evidence is arguably the most important step in conducting a high-quality systematic review. In a human research study, selection of the appropriate group to be studied is widely understood to be

BOX 4-2
Prevention Topics with Insufficient Evidence
for One or More Population Subgroups

- Behavioral counseling in primary care to promote a healthy diet
- Behavioral counseling in primary care to promote physical activity
- Breast-feeding
- Counseling to prevent skin cancer
- Counseling to prevent tobacco use and tobacco-caused disease
- Interventions in primary care to reduce alcohol misuse
- Lung cancer screening
- Newborn hearing screening
- Prevention of dental caries in preschool-age children
- Primary care interventions to prevent low back pain in adults
- Routine vitamin supplementation to prevent cancer and cardiovascular disease
- Screening and behavioral counseling
- Screening and interventions for overweight in children and adolescents
- Screening for bacterial vaginosis in pregnancy
- Screening for breast cancer
- Screening for cervical cancer
- Screening for chlamydial infection
- Screening for coronary heart disease
- Screening for dementia
- Screening for depression
- Screening for family and intimate partner violence
- Screening for gestational diabetes mellitus
- Screening for glaucoma
- Screening for gonorrhea
- Screening for hepatitis C in adults
- Screening for high blood pressure
- Screening for lipid disorders in adults
- Screening for obesity in adults
- Screening for oral cancer
- Screening for prostate cancer
- Screening for skin cancer
- Screening for suicide risk
- Screening for thyroid disease
- Screening for Type II diabetes mellitus in adults

NOTE: Each clinical topic or preventive service that the USPSTF has reviewed may lead to one or more separate population-specific recommendations. The USPSTF rates the strength of its recommendations as "I" for "insufficient" when evidence on whether the service is effective is lacking, of poor quality, or conflicting and the balance of benefits and harms cannot be determined. In such cases, the USPSTF does not recommend either for or against the routine provision of the service. For the topics listed here, there was at least one population subgroup with an "I" rating.
SOURCE: AHRQ (2006).

critical to obtaining valid findings. The comparable step in a systematic review is the identification of all relevant studies meeting the eligibility criteria for the review. A comprehensive search is necessary because there is no way of knowing whether the missing studies are missing at random or missing for a reason critical to understanding current knowledge.

Minimizing Bias

Bias—which is the tendency for a study to produce results that depart systematically from the truth—is the biggest threat to the validity of a review.[9] Box 4-3 describes the potential sources of bias in the individual studies identified during the search for evidence and in the review itself.

Without the use of systematic methods to guard against bias in the review, useless or harmful interventions may appear to be worthwhile and beneficial interventions may appear to be useless (Chalmers, 2003). Reporting biases have important implications during the search for evidence. For example, it is now well established that positive results are more likely to be published than null or negative results both for entire studies (Dickersin, 2005; Dickersin and Min, 1993) and for selected outcomes (Chan et al., 2004). Furthermore, a growing literature indicates that industry-sponsored research is more likely to favor the industry sponsor's product than non-industry-sponsored research (Als-Nielsen et al., 2003; Bekelman et al., 2003; Heres et al., 2006; Jorgensen et al., 2006; Lexchin et al., 2003; Peppercorn et al., 2007).

Studies have also found that the direction of the results (i.e., positive or negative) can be associated with the language of publication (Egger et al., 1997), the impact factor[10] of the journal (Easterbrook et al., 1991), and publication in the "gray literature" (Hopewell et al., 2007b), for example, research abstracts, government reports, and theses. Publication biases also relate to where a study is published, as some sources are more accessible than others. Some systematic reviewers find it difficult to readily identify studies published in non-English-language journals, the gray literature, and certain specialty journals.

One favorable development is that the rate of universal registration of RCTs is growing. This development may help address the publication bias related to studies of this design (World Health Organizations, 2007). Unfortunately, there is no similar organized effort to promote the registration of observational studies.

---

[9]Elsewhere in this report, the term "bias" is used to refer to bias due to conflicts of interest.

[10]The "impact factor" is a commonly used ratio developed to estimate the relative impact or influence of biomedical journals (Garfield, 2006).

BOX 4-3
Sources of Bias in Individual Studies and Systematic Reviews

Biases can lead to under-estimation or over-estimation of a true intervention effect. Systematic reviews should be based on the best evidence available to answer the questions posed, controlling against systematic bias both in the individual studies and in the review itself.

The key types of bias that can affect the internal validity of individual studies are as follows:

- **Selection bias**—systematic differences between comparison groups in a study, for example, in a clinical trial if patients assigned to the treatment group have a better prognosis than those assigned to the placebo group.
- **Attrition bias**—systematic differences in withdrawals from a study or exclusions from the study results between the study's comparison groups.
- **Performance bias**—systematic differences in care, apart from the intervention being evaluated or the measurement of exposure, provided to different comparison groups in a study.
- **Detection bias**—systematic differences in outcome assessment or verification in comparison groups (also called "ascertainment bias").
- **Within-study reporting bias**—systematic differences between reported and unreported findings.

The key types of bias that may affect the validity of a systematic review are as follows:

- **Reporting bias**—systematic differences may exist between reported and non-reported studies (e.g., a higher proportion of studies with positive findings than studies with null or negative findings may be published ["publication bias"]). Systematic differences in findings may also exist between MEDLINE-indexed and non-MEDLINE-indexed journals, English-language and non-English-language publications (language bias), easier and harder-to-access literature (e.g., null or negative findings are published in journals with less of an impact or in the "gray literature"), and studies with commercial funding sources.
- **Information bias**—key details about the study may be missing, particularly for studies that appear in the literature only as abstracts, which are subject to reporting bias.

SOURCES: Dickersin (2002); Higgins and Green (2006); West et al. (2002).

Sources of Evidence

Most systematic reviewers limit their searches to electronic databases, for reasons of time, convenience, expense, and their own limitations in knowledge and understanding of the appropriate review methodology.

In the United States, most reviews include a search of the MEDLINE[11] database; and fewer include searches of the Cochrane Central Register of Controlled Trials, EMBASE,[12] CINHAL,[13] the Web of Science, the Latin American Caribbean Health Sciences Literature (LILACS), and other databases.

A search of just one electronic database is likely to identify only a subset of all relevant studies for inclusion in a review. Early research showed that searches of the MEDLINE database for clinical trials identified only about 50 percent of all relevant trials (Dickersin et al., 1985, 1994). This led to a modification of the MEDLINE indexing system to include methodology indexing terms, and the Cochrane Collaboration further enhanced the ability to retrieve relevant information by contributing trials that it had identified to a central repository (Dickersin et al., 2002).

Researchers at McMaster University and elsewhere have extensively tested search strategies to determine those strategies that are optimal for detecting reports on RCTs and other types of studies used in systematic reviews (Wieland and Dickersin, 2005; Wilczynski et al., 2005). However, more research is needed to determine the best search strategy for identifying adverse effects, for example, by using evidence from nonrandomized studies when one is examining adverse effects. Some studies suggest that because highly sensitive searches tend to yield large numbers of irrelevant studies, there should be a greater emphasis on improving both reporting and indexing to facilitate the conduct of systematic reviews (Golder et al., 2006; Wieland and Dickersin, 2005).

Hand searches   Although many reviewers also conduct a hand search[14] of reference lists and other review articles, few hand searches include conference proceedings or recent issues of key journals. Because only about half of all results reported in conference proceedings are ultimately reported in key journals (Scherer et al., 2007) and only full publication is associated with

---

[11]MEDLINE is the United States National Library of Medicine's bibliographic database of the literature from medicine, nursing, dentistry, veterinary medicine, allied health, and preclinical sciences. See http://www.nlm.nih.gov for more information.

[12]Excerpta Medica (EMBASE) is a biomedical and pharmaceutical database indexing over 3,500 international journals in drug research, pharmacology, pharmaceutics, toxicology, clinical and experimental human medicine, health policy and management, public health, occupational health, environmental health, drug dependence and abuse, psychiatry, forensic medicine, and biomedical engineering/instrumentation. See http://www.embase.com/ for more information.

[13]Cumulative Index to Nursing & Allied Health Literature (CINHAL) covers literature related to nursing and allied health from 1982 to the present. See http://www.cinahl.com/prodsvcs/cinahldb.htm for more information.

[14]A hand search is a manual review of each page of selected individual journals published during a specified period.

positive findings, those conducting systematic reviews may indicate that a treatment is successful when it actually is not, if abstracts from conference proceedings are not included and hand searches are not done. Adding to this potential bias is the fact that the information in abstracts is limited at best, making it difficult to judge the validity of study methods and results.

In a recent systematic review of 34 studies comparing the sensitivity of hand searches with that of electronic searches, Hopewell and colleagues (2007a) found that hand searches identified 92 to 100 percent of the total number of reports of randomized trials. In contrast, electronic searches had a lower yield; a search of the MEDLINE database retrieved 55 percent of the total reports, a search of EMBASE retrieved 49 percent, and a search of PsycINFO retrieved 67 percent.

Step 4: Critically Appraise the Evidence

A properly conducted systematic review systematically scrutinizes and documents the quality, strength, and consistency of the studies that make up the relevant body of evidence (Box 4-4). The quality of an individual study relates to all aspects of its design and execution, including the extent to which bias is avoided or minimized. Each individual study, including past systematic reviews (if they are available), should be meticulously examined to identify whether the study incorporated methods that protect against bias and how the various types of bias may have affected the results (Khan and Kleijnen, 2001). Both experimental and observational studies must also be judged for their external validity or for their applicability to the population of interest. Without a thorough analysis of the body of research, the review will not meet decision makers' need to know which evidence is valid, for whom it is valid, and under what circumstances it is valid.

Despite the imperative for the use of standardized methods in systematic reviews, current practices appear to fall short of expectations. This is particularly worrisome because end users—patients, clinicians, and others—may accept the findings in published reviews at face value. Deficiencies are commonplace; for example, the methods may be poorly documented or poorly executed, the quality of individual studies may not be assessed or described, inappropriate statistical methods may have been used, and errors in the analyses may not be identified (Bhandari et al., 2001; Delaney et al., 2005; Glenny et al., 2003; Hayden et al., 2006; Jadad and McQuay, 1996; Jadad et al., 2000; Mallen et al., 2006; Moher et al., 2007; Shea et al., 2002; Whiting et al., 2005). The following describes examples of recent findings.

Moher and colleagues (2007) assessed the quality of 300 systematic reviews identified through a MEDLINE search for English-language reviews. Most of the reviews (213 of 300) concerned therapeutic or preven-

---

BOX 4-4
Key Concepts in Appraising Evidence

Assessing the effectiveness of a health intervention requires careful scrutiny of the quality, strength, and consistency of the individual and systematic reviews that make up the relevant body of evidence. These and other related concepts are defined below:

- **Study quality**—For an individual study, study quality refers to all aspects of a study's design and execution and the extent to which bias is avoided or minimized. A related concept is internal validity, that is, the degree to which the results of a study are likely to be true and free of bias.
- **Strength of findings**—The strength of the findings can refer to those of a single study or a body of evidence. The term can be used to refer to the numbers of participants and events observed (greater strength for greater numbers), as well as to the magnitude of the effect, either beneficial or harmful.
- **Consistency**—Consistency refers to a body of evidence in which individual studies report similar findings, even though there might be some variations in the populations studied or the forms or dosages of the interventions.
- **External validity**—External validity (or applicability) refers to the extent to which the effects observed in a research study can be applied to a real-life population and setting.
- **Estimate of effect**—The estimate of the effect is the relationship observed between an intervention and an outcome. In intervention studies, the estimate of effect may be expressed as the study effect size, relative risk, risk difference, an odds ratio, the number needed to treat, or some other measure of effect or association.

SOURCES: GRADE Working Group (2004); Ioannidis and Lau (2004); Khan et al. (2001a,b); Treadwell et al. (2006); West et al. (2002).

---

tive interventions and were published in specialty journals (272 of 300). The authors found that only 11 percent of the reviews were based on a standard protocol, less than one-quarter (23 percent) considered or assessed publication bias, and 41 percent did not report their funding sources. The reviews searched a median of three electronic databases and two other sources. There was little consistency in how the electronic searches were documented in the reviews; only 69 percent of the reviews reported the years of publication searched.

Mallen and colleagues (2006) examined how 78 English-language systematic reviews analyzed the quality of the original observational studies. All the reviews were published in peer-reviewed journals from 2003 to 2004. The reviews of the Cochrane Collaboration and United Kingdom

National Health Service R&D Health Technology Assessment Programme (HTA)[15] were excluded because they were known to include formal quality assessment procedures. In 36 of the 78 reviews, the quality of the individual studies was not assessed. Although the quality of the studies was reported in 39 reviews, the reviews used 10 different quality assessment techniques, making it difficult to compare them. It was unknown whether quality was assessed for three of the reviews.

Investigators have also identified data extraction errors in many systematic reviews, including Cochrane Collaboration and other standards-based reviews (Gøtzsche et al., 2007; Jones et al., 2005). Some errors could be averted by using a second extractor. For example, in preparation for a systematic review of the use of melatonin for the management of sleep disorders, a Canadian team found that more errors were made by using single extraction with verification by a second person than with double data extraction (Buscemi et al., 2006).

Hierarchies of Evidence

Organizations that develop clinical guidelines, as well as other reviewers of evidence, often look to hierarchies of evidence to gauge the relative strength of individual studies. The hierarchies provide frameworks that assign types of evidence (e.g., RCTs, controlled trials without randomization, and well-designed case series or cohort studies) to various levels, each with a corresponding grade. Numerous hierarchies and typologies have proliferated—each with its own system of letters, codes, and symbols (Schünemann et al., 2003). As Table 4-5 illustrates, the end result is greater confusion rather than clarification.[16]

Hierarchies that include systematic reviews typically place them above single studies of the same design. Montori and colleagues (2003) explained that systematic reviews of RCTs should be at the top of the hierarchy for intervention questions because of their emphasis on methodological quality and, if a meta-analysis is employed, the availability of more precise estimates of the association or treatment effect.

Evidence hierarchies have helped raise awareness that some study designs are less subject to bias than others (Glasziou et al., 2004). Hierarchies, however, consider just the type of research study (e.g., RCTs or prospective observational studies) and not the quality of the individual studies (Poolman et al., 2006). Findings from a poorly conducted trial should not

---

[15]HTA reviews are systematic reviews conducted under the auspices of the United Kingdom National Health Service R&D Health Technology Assessment Programme.

[16]Table 5-2 in Chapter 5 illustrates the confusion in evidence hierarchies and recommendation grades in cardiology.

TABLE 4-5 Selected Examples of Evidence Hierarchies for Three Cardiology Interventions

Intervention and Organization	Quality of the Evidence	Type of Evidence
Oral anticoagulation therapy in patients with atrial fibrillation and rheumatic mitral valve disease		
American Heart Association	Level B	Single randomized trial or nonrandomized studies
Scottish Intercollegiate Guidelines Network	Level 4	Expert opinion
American College of Chest Physicians	Grade C+	No RCTs (but strong RCT results can be unequivocally extrapolated) or overwhelming evidence from observational studies
Implantable cardioverter-defibrillator for cardiac arrest due to sustained ventricular fibrillation or ventricular tachycardia		
American College of Cardiology/ American Heart Association	Level A	Multiple RCTs or meta-analyses
Scottish Intercollegiate Guidelines Network	Level 3/4	Nonanalytic studies, e.g., case reports and case series
European Society of Cardiology	Level B	Single RCT or large nonrandomized studies
Carotid endarterectomy for internal carotid artery stenosis or symptomatic stenosis		
American College of Cardiology/ American Heart Association	Level C	Consensus opinion of experts, results of case studies, or standard of care
American Academy of Neurology	Class I/II	Class I = prospective RCT with masked outcome assessment, in a representative population* Class II = prospective matched group cohort study in a representative population with masked outcome assessment that meets all four Class I criteria (a to d) or an RCT in a representative population that lacks one of the Class I criteria
Veterans Health Administration	Level I	At least one properly conducted randomized controlled trial

*The following are also required: (a) primary outcome(s) clearly defined; (b) exclusion and inclusion criteria clearly defined; (c) adequate accounting for dropouts and crossovers with numbers sufficiently low to have a minimal potential for bias; and (d) relevant baseline characteristics are presented and are substantially equivalent among treatment groups or there is an appropriate statistical adjustment for the differences.

SOURCE: NGC (2007); Schünemann et al. (2003).

necessarily trump evidence from a nonrandomized study. All the evidence that is found should be clearly described and scrutinized and not just assigned to a level of a hierarchy (Glasziou et al., 2004).

Step 5: Synthesize the Body of Evidence

The core of a systematic review is a concise and transparent synthesis of the results of the studies included in the review. The language of the review should be simple and clear so that it is usable and accessible to decision makers. The synthesis may be purely qualitative; quantitative but only descriptive, in that study results are presented in a common metric but not combined; or it may be complemented by a meta-analysis that combines the individual study results and allows statistical inference.

There are no standard guidelines for conducting or presenting the synthesis. However, the Cochrane Collaboration produces and regularly updates a methods handbook for Cochrane reviews of clinical trials that is available on the Internet (Higgins and Green, 2006). The AHRQ Effective Health Care Program is currently developing a methods manual for systematic reviews that focuses on comparative effectiveness (AHRQ, 2007a).

The synthesis should collate, describe, and summarize the following key features of the individual studies that could have a bearing on the findings:

- Characteristics of the patient population, the care setting, and type of provider
- Intervention (route, dose, timing, duration)
- Comparison group
- Outcome measures and timing of assessments
- Quality of the evidence (i.e., risk of bias) from individual studies and possible influence on findings
- Sample sizes
- Quantitative results and analyses including examination of whether the study estimates of effect are consistent across studies
- Examination of potential sources of study heterogeneity, if relevant

The investigators should consider carefully if a meta-analysis is appropriate and should combine clinical judgment and a thorough understanding of the individual studies with the aggregated result. A summary estimate has the potential to mislead and lead to spurious conclusions (Editors, 2005). A detailed description of meta-analysis is beyond the scope of this report; however, an excellent review of the analytic considerations in conducting meta-analyses can be found in the text *Methods for Meta-Analysis in Medical Research* (Sutton et al., 2000).

The synthesis should not include policy recommendations. If the systematic review is both scientific and transparent, decision makers should be able to interpret the evidence, to know what is not known, and to describe the extent to which the evidence is applicable to clinical practice and particular subgroups of patients (Santaguida et al., 2005). Making evidence-based decisions—such as when a guideline developer recommends what should and should not be done in specific clinical circumstances—is a distinct and separate process from conducting a systematic review and is the subject of the next chapter.

Journal Standards for Reporting Systematic Reviews

In the past decade, researchers, clinicians, epidemiologists, statisticians, and editors have collaborated to develop standards for the reporting of findings from clinical trials and meta-analyses of randomized and nonrandomized studies in journals. The collaboration arose from concerns that study quality was poorly reflected in the manuscripts that present study findings. Table 4-6 describes the basic requirements of these three standardized reporting formats, Consolidated Standards for Reporting Trials (CONSORT), Quality of Reporting of Meta-analyses (QUOROM)[17] for RCTs, and Meta-analysis Of Observational Studies in Epidemiology (MOOSE). Other approaches to standardized reporting including Strengthening the Reporting of Observational Studies in Epidemiology (STROBE) and Standards for Reporting of Diagnostic Accuracy (STARD) (Bossuyt et al., 2003; Ebrahim and Clarke, 2007; von Elm et al., 2007).

CONSORT uses standardized checklists and a flow diagram to ensure the proper and consistent reporting of the benefits and harms reported from RCTs (Ioannidis et al., 2004; Moher et al., 2001b). Since its publication in 1996, many journals have adopted CONSORT, and as a result, the quality of reporting of the findings from RCTs has improved substantially (Moher et al., 2001a,b, 2007).

After the release of CONSORT, two standard formats for reporting on meta-analyses were developed: QUOROM for meta-analyses of RCTs and MOOSE for meta-analyses of observational studies (Moher et al., 1999; Stroup et al., 2000). Like CONSORT, QUOROM and MOOSE use checklists to ensure that meta-analyses include sections describing the background, search strategy, methods, results, a discussion, and conclusions. However, as Table 4-7 indicates, the use of QUOROM and MOOSE is not widely required by most prominent journals, according to the instructions

---

[17]QUOROM standards are currently being updated under the name PRISMA (Preferred Reporting Items for Systematic Reviews and Meta-Analyses).

TABLE 4-6 Comparison of Reporting Standards in CONSORT, QUOROM, and MOOSE

| System, Study Type | Required Information | | | | |
	Title and Abstract	Introduction	Methods	Results	Discussion
CONSORT, trials	For the abstract, identify the method of selection of participants	Scientific background and explanation of rationale	Participants, interventions, objectives, outcomes, sample size, randomization, blinding, and statistical methods	Participant flow, recruitment, baseline data, numbers analyzed, outcomes and estimation, ancillary analyses, and adverse events	Interpretation, generalizability, overall evidence
QUOROM, meta-analyses of trials	For the title, identify the report as a meta-analysis (or a systematic review) of RCTs; for the abstract, use a structured abstract format that describes the objectives, data sources, review methods, results, and conclusions	Clinical problem, biological rationale for the intervention, and rationale for review	Searching, selection, validity assessment, data abstraction, study characteristics, quantitative data, and synthesis	Trial flow, study characteristics, and quantitative data synthesis	Key findings, clinical inferences, interpretation of results, potential biases, and future research agenda
MOOSE, meta-analyses of observational studies	For the abstract, identify the type of study and use structured abstract	Clinical problem, hypothesis, outcome of study, exposure or intervention used, study design used, and study population	Search strategy, qualification of searchers, software and databases used, potential biases, rationale for studies and selection of data used, assessment of confounding, study quality and heterogeneity, and statistical methods	Graph and table summarizing the results, sensitivity testing, and indication of the statistical uncertainty of the findings	Assessment of bias, justification of exclusion, quality of studies included, alternative explanation, generalization, future research, and funding source

TABLE 4-7 Use of Reporting Standards in Leading Biomedical Journals

Journal	Standards Are Specifically Mentioned in the Journal's Instructions to Authors			ICMJE Uniform Requirements Are Included in the Journal's Instructions to Authors	
	CONSORT (1996)	QUOROM (1999)	MOOSE (2000)	Entire manuscript	Selected sections of manuscript
Annals of Internal Medicine	✓	✓	✓	✓	
Archives of General Psychiatry	✓			✓	
British Medical Journal	✓	✓	✓	✓	
CANCER	✓				✓
CHEST	✓			✓	
Circulation	✓		✓		✓
Diabetes					✓
Hypertension	✓			✓	
JAMA	✓	✓	✓	✓	
Journal of Clinical Oncology	✓				✓
Journal of the National Cancer Institute	✓			✓	
Lancet	✓			✓	
New England Journal of Medicine	✓			✓	
Obstetrics and Gynecology	✓	✓	✓		
Pediatrics	✓			✓	
Radiology	✓	✓			✓
Reviews in Clinical Gerontology					
Spine	✓			✓	

NOTE: For systematic reviews, the International Committee of Medical Journal Editors (ICMJE) encourages but does not require authors to consult the QUOROM and MOOSE reporting guidelines; for RCTs, the use of the CONSORT reporting guidelines is required.
SOURCES: Annals of Internal Medicine (2007); Archives of General Psychiatry (2007); British Medical Journal (2007); CANCER (2007); CHEST (2006); Circulation (2007); Diabetes (2007); Hypertension (2007); ICMJE (2006); JAMA (2007); Journal of Clinical Oncology (2007); Journal of the National Cancer Institute (2007); Lancet (2007); New England Journal of Medicine (2007); Obstetrics and Gynecology (2007); Pediatrics (2007); Radiology (2007); Reviews in Clinical Gerontology (2007); Spine (2007).

for authors that they publish. Appendix D provides the QUOROM and MOOSE formats.

RECOMMENDATIONS

As noted earlier, this chapter's recommendations are intended to guide the conduct of systematic reviews produced under the aegis of a national clinical effectiveness assessment program ("the Program"). The recommendations draw from the research examined in this chapter and are based on the consensus of the committee. The Program must address three critical challenges: (1) the development or endorsement of standards to ensure high-quality and usable evidence reviews, (2) methods research to find solutions to the technical challenges of systematic review, and (3) a research workforce that is sufficient to meet the Program's demands.

Standards

Systematic reviews of evidence on the effectiveness of health care services provide a central link between the generation of research and clinical decision making. Systematic review is itself a science and, in fact, is a new and dynamic science with evolving methods. In the United States, much can be gained by beginning to systemize and standardize the generation of systematic reviews as soon as possible. At a minimum, this should include standard reporting formats and common terminology for characterizing the strength of the evidence in order to ensure that evidence reviews are accessible and usable for all types of decision makers.

Under the status quo, the quality of published reviews is variable and often unreliable. Judging the quality of reviews is difficult at best because the methods used to produce the reviews are so frequently poorly documented. The numerous grading schemes and hierarchies that are used are confusing. An overreliance on hierarchies is also inappropriate because such hierarchies fail to account for the quality of the underlying research. Reporting standards exist, but are often not used or enforced.

Recommendation: The Program should develop evidence-based, methodologic standards for systematic reviews, including a common language for characterizing the strength of evidence. The Program should fund reviewers only if they commit to and consistently meet these standards.

- **The Program should invest in advancing the scientific methods underlying the conduct of systematic reviews and, when appropriate, update the standards for the reviews it funds.**

Methods

Investing in the science of research synthesis will increase the quality and the value of the evidence provided in systematic reviews. As a new field, attention to the methods used to conduct systematic reviews and attention to improving the existing methods are critically important. About two decades of research underpins the methods that are being used to search, identify, appraise, and interpret the evidence presented in a systematic review (Egger et al., 2001; Mulrow and Lohr, 2001). Much remains to be learned, and numerous unresolved methodological issues remain (Helfand, 2005; Neumann, 2006). Research is needed on methods for identifying observational studies, using observational evidence in the absence of randomized data, and better understanding the impact of potential biases (Egger et al., 2003; Gluud, 2006; Hopewell et al., 2007a,b; Kunz et al., 2007; Song et al., 2000). Box 4-5 lists some of the most pressing methodological issues.

Recommendation: The Program should assess the capacity of the research workforce to meet the Program's needs, and, if deemed appropriate, it should expand training opportunities in systematic review and comparative effectiveness research methods.

Research Workforce

It is not known how many researchers in the United States are adequately trained and qualified to conduct systematic reviews on the effectiveness of health care services. At present, AHRQ provides predoctoral and postdoctoral educational and career development grants in health services research (Medicare Payment Advisory Commission, 2007). The agency also provides institution-level grants to support the planning and development of health services research in certain types of institutions. The NIH also supports a wide range of research training opportunities. However, it is not known to what extent the AHRQ and NIH training programs focus on systematic reviews.

Thus, it is unknown but likely that the nation has insufficient human capacity to support an expanded national effort to generate systematic reviews of clinical effectiveness. The Program should assess the research workforce to see if it is adequate. If necessary, the Program should provide more opportunities for training in the conduct of systematic reviews and comparative effectiveness research. A field can grow and produce high-quality work only if it attracts and retains creative investigators. There must be opportunities to learn and grow professionally. To be attractive to the best and the brightest individuals, the field must adhere to high standards of research quality and scientific integrity, be open to new ideas and people,

---

BOX 4-5
Unresolved Methodological Issues in
Conducting Systematic Reviews

Locating and Selecting Studies
- How best to identify all relevant published studies
- Whether to include and how best to identify non-English-language studies
- Whether to include and how best to identify unpublished studies and studies in the gray literature (e.g., abstracts)
- Search strategies for identifying observational studies in MEDLINE, EMBASE, and other databases
- Search strategies for identifying studies of diagnostic accuracy in MEDLINE, EMBASE, and other databases

Assessing Study Quality
- Understanding the sources of reporting deficiencies in studies being synthesized
- Understanding and identifying potential biases and conflicts of interest
- Quality thresholds for study inclusion and the management of individual study quality in the context of a review

Collecting Data
- Identifying and selecting information to assess treatment harms
- Obtaining important unpublished data from relevant studies
- Methods used for data abstraction

Analyzing and Presenting Results
- Use of qualitative data in systematic reviews
- Use of economic data in systematic reviews
- Methods for combining results of diagnostic test accuracy

Statistical Methods (e.g., statistical heterogeneity, fixed versus random effects, and meta-regression)
- Inclusion of interstudy variability into displays of results
- How best to display findings and their reliability for users
- Methods and validity of indirect comparisons

Interpreting Results
- Understanding why reviews on similar topics may yield different results
- Updating systematic reviews
- Frequency of updates

SOURCE: Cochrane Collaboration (2007); Higgins and Green (2006).

---

and provide excitement about the potential to contribute to health research and to health care practice overall. Moreover, the academic community must recognize the scientific scholarship that is required to conduct high-quality systematic reviews.

OTHER PROGRAM CHALLENGES

Keeping Reviews Up-to-Date

Systematic reviews are not only difficult and time consuming, they also must be kept up-to-date to ensure patient safety. Having an organization that exercises oversight on the production of systematic reviews, for example, the Cochrane Collaboration or professional societies that produce clinical practice guidelines, provides an infrastructure and chain of responsibility for the updating of reviews. There has been little research on updating, and the research that does exist indicates that not all organizations have mechanisms for systematically updating their reviews.

In 2001, Shekelle and colleagues (2001) examined how quickly the AHRQ guidelines went out of date. At the time of that study, they classified only 3 of the 17 guidelines in circulation at that time as still valid. About half of the guidelines were out of date in 5.8 years from the time of their release, and at 3.6 years, at least 10 percent were out of date. A more recent report examining a sample of 100 high-quality systematic reviews of interventions found that within 5.5 years, half of the reviews had new evidence that would substantively change the conclusions about the effectiveness of interventions, and within 2 years almost 25 percent had such evidence (Shojania et al., 2007). The frequency of updating was associated with the clinical topic area and the initial heterogeneity of the results.

Thus, it appears that the failure to update systematic reviews and guidelines within a few years could easily result in patient care that is not evidence based and, worse, care that is not as effective as possible or potentially dangerous.

New and Emerging Technologies

Although this chapter has focused on comprehensive, systematic reviews, the committee recognizes that some decision makers have a legitimate need for objective advisories on new and emerging technologies in order to respond to coverage requests when few, if any, high-quality studies or systematic reviews exist. In addition, patients and providers want information on new health care services as soon as the services become known, often because manufacturers are pressing them to adopt a product or because patients have read direct-to-consumer advertising and want answers from their physicians and other health care providers.

Private technology assessment organizations, such as the ECRI Institute and Hayes, Inc., have responded to the market demand for early reviews of new technologies (ECRI, 2006b; Hayes, Inc., 2007). These firms and other private, proprietary organizations offer clients brief reviews based on readily available sources of information. Two examples are provided in Appendix E (as proprietary products, they are not in the public domain). The reviews aggregate what little is known from searches of electronic databases (e.g., MEDLINE, EMBASE, or the Cochrane Central Register of Controlled Trials) and published conference abstracts. Other easily obtained information, such as reports from FDA advisory committee meetings, may also be included. Typically, the reviews include a brief description of an intervention; its relevance to clinical care; a short, preliminary list of the relevant research citations that have been identified; two- to three-paragraph summaries of selected research abstracts; and details on the methods used to search the literature.

The Program should consider producing brief advisories on new and emerging technologies in addition to full systematic reviews. If so, like the ECRI Institute and Hayes, Inc., products, the advisories produced under the aegis of the Program should clearly emphasize and highlight the limitations of the information. The advisories clearly state their limitations, so that no one will misinterpret them as an adequate substitute for substantive assessments of evidence on effectiveness.

REFERENCES

AHRQ (Agency for Healthcare Research and Quality). 2006. *The guide to clinical preventive services 2006: Recommendations of the U.S. Preventive Services Task Force. AHRQ. Pub. No. 06-0588.* Rockville, MD: AHRQ.

———. 2007a. *Guide for conducting comparative effectiveness reviews (Draft for public comment)* http://effectivehealthcare.ahrq.gov/getInvolved/commentFormMethodsGuide. cfm?DocID=1 (accessed October 10, 2007).

———. 2007b. *User's guide to registries evaluating patient outcomes: Summary. AHRQ Pub. No. 07-EHC001-2.* Rockville, MD: AHRQ.

AHRQ EPC Program (Evidence-based Practice Center Program). 2007. *Template for submissions of topics for AHRQ evidence reports or technology assessments* http://www.ahrq. gov/clinic/epcpartner/epcesubtempl.doc (accessed January 17, 2007).

Allen, C., and M. Clarke. 2007 (unpublished). *International activity in Cochrane Review Groups with a focus on the USA.* Cochrane Collaboration.

Als-Nielsen, B., W. Chen, C. Gluud, and L. L. Kjaergard. 2003. Association of funding and conclusions in randomized drug trials: A reflection of treatment effect or adverse events? *JAMA* 290(7):921-928.

Annals of Internal Medicine. 2007. *Information for authors* http://www.annals.org/shared/ author_info.html (accessed July 11, 2007).

Antman, E. M., J. Lau, B. Kupelnick, F. Mosteller, and T. C. Chalmers. 1992. A comparison of meta-analyses of randomized control trials and recommendations of clinical experts. Treatments for myocardial infarction. *JAMA* 268(2):240-248.

Archives of General Psychiatry. 2007. *Instructions for authors* http://archpsyc.ama-assn.org/ misc/ifora.dtl (accessed July 12, 2007).

Atkins, D. 2007. Creating and synthesizing evidence with decision makers in mind: Integrating evidence from clinical trials and other study designs. *Medical Care* 45(10 Suppl 2): S16-S22.

Atkins, D., K. Fink, and J. Slutsky. 2005. Better information for better health care: The Evidence-based Practice Center program and the Agency for Healthcare Research and Quality. *Annals of Internal Medicine* 142(12 Part 2):1035-1041.

Barton, M. 2007. *Using systematic reviews to develop clinical recommendations (Submitted responses to the IOM HECS committee meeting, January 25, 2007)*. Washington, DC.

BCBSA (Blue Cross and Blue Shield Association). 2007. *Blue Cross and Blue Shield Association proposes payer-funded institute to evaluate what medical treatments work best* http://www.bcbs.com/news/bcbsa/blue-cross-and-blue-shield-association-proposes-payer-funded-institute.html (accessed May 2007).

Bekelman, J. E., Y. Li, and C. P. Gross. 2003. Scope and impact of financial conflicts of interest in biomedical research: A systematic review. *JAMA* 289(4):454-465.

Bhandari, M., F. Morrow, A. V. Kulkarni, and P. Tornetta. 2001. Meta-analyses in orthopaedic surgery: A systematic review of their methodologies. *Journal of Bone and Joint Surgery* 83A:15-24.

Bossuyt, P. M., J. B. Reitsma, D. E. Bruns, C. A. Gatsonis, P. P. Glasziou, L. M. Irwig, D. Moher, D. Rennie, H. C. de Vet, and J. G. Lijmer. 2003. The STARD statement for reporting studies of diagnostic accuracy: Explanation and elaboration. *Clinical Chemistry* 49:7-18.

British Medical Journal. 2007. *Resources for authors: Article requirements* http://resources.bmj.com/bmj/authors/article-submission/article-requirements (accessed July 11, 2007).

Buscemi, N., L. Hartling, B. Vandermeer, L. Tjosvold, and T. P. Klassen. 2006. Single data extraction generated more errors than double data extraction in systematic reviews. *Journal of Clinical Epidemiology* 59(7):697-703.

CANCER. 2007. *CANCER instructions for authors* http://www.interscience.wiley.com/cancer/ (accessed July 11, 2007).

CDC (Centers for Disease Control and Prevention). 2007. *Community preventive services: Methods: Effectiveness evaluation* http://www.thecommunityguide.org/methods/ (accessed October 3, 2007).

Chalmers, I. 2003. Trying to do more good than harm in policy and practice: The role of rigorous, transparent, up-to-date evaluations. *Annals of the American Academy of Political and Social Science* 589(1):22-40.

———. 2005. Academia's failure to support systematic reviews. *Lancet* 365(9458):469.

Chalmers, I., and D. G. Altman. 1995. *Systematic reviews.* London: BMJ Publications.

Chalmers, I., J. Hetherington, and M. Newdick. 1986. The Oxford database of perinatal trials: Developing a register of published reports of controlled trials. *Controlled Clinical Trials* 7(4):306-324.

Chalmers, I., M. Enkin, and M. Keirse. 1989. *Effective care in pregnancy and childbirth.* Oxford, UK: Oxford University Press.

Chan, A. W., A. Hrobjartsson, M. T. Haahr, P. C. Gøtzsche, and D. G. Altman. 2004. Emperical evidence for selective reporting of outcomes in randomized trials: Comparison of protocols to published articles. *JAMA* 291:2457-2465.

CHEST. 2006. *CHEST instructions to authors and statement of CHEST policies* http://www.chestjournal.org/misc/PolicyInstruxA.pdf (accessed July 11, 2007).

Chou, R., and M. Helfand. 2005. Challenges in systematic reviews that assess treatment harms. *Annals of Internal Medicine* 142(12 Part 2):1090-1099.

Circulation. 2007. *Instructions for authors* http://circ.ahajournals.org/misc/ifora.shtml (accessed July 12, 2007).

Claxton, K., J. T. Cohen, and P. J. Neumann. 2005. When is evidence sufficient? *Health Affairs* 24(1):93-101.

Cochrane Collaboration. 2007. *Methods groups newsletter* Vol. 11. Oxford, UK.

Congressional Budget Office. 2007. Research on the comparative effectiveness of medical treatments: Options for an expanded federal role. *Testimony by Director Peter R. Orszag before House Ways and Means Subcommittee on Health* http://www.cbo.gov/ftpdocs/82xx/doc8209/Comparative_Testimony.pdf (accessed June 12, 2007).

Cook, D. J., C. D. Mulrow, and R. B. Haynes. 1997. Systematic reviews: Synthesis of best evidence for clinical decisions. *Annals of Internal Medicine* 126(5):376-380.

Cooper, H. M., and R. Rosenthal. 1980. A comparison of statistical and traditional procedures for summarizing research. *Psychological Bulletin* 87:442-449.

Counsell, C. 1997. Formulating questions and locating primary studies for inclusion in systematic reviews. *Annals of Internal Medicine* 127(5):380-387.

Delaney, A., S. M. Bagshaw, A. Ferland, B. Manns, and K. B. Laupland. 2005. A systematic evaluation of the quality of meta-analyses in the critical care literature. *Critical Care* 9:R575-R582.

Diabetes. 2007. *Diabetes instructions for authors* http://care.diabetesjournals.org/misc/ifora.shtml (accessed July 30, 2007).

Dickersin, K. 2002. Systematic reviews in epidemiology: Why are we so far behind? *International Journal of Epidemiology* 31(1):6-12.

———. 2005. Publication bias: Recognizing the problem, understanding its origins and scope, and preventing harm. In *Publication bias in meta-analysis: Prevention, assessment, and adjustments*. Edited by Rothstein, H., A. Sutton, and M. Borenstein. London, UK: John Wiley and Sons, Ltd.

———. 2007 (unpublished). *Steps in evidence-based healthcare*. PowerPoint Presentation. Baltimore, MD.

Dickersin, K., and Y.-I. Min. 1993. Publication bias: The problem that won't go away. In *Doing more good than harm: The evaluation of health care interventions*. Edited by Warren, K. S., and F. Mosteller. New York: New York Academy of Sciences. Pp. 135-148.

Dickersin, K., and E. Manheimer. 1998. The Cochrane Collaboration: Evaluation of health care and services using systematic reviews of the results of randomized controlled trials. *Clinical Obstetrics and Gynecology* 41(2):315-331.

Dickersin, K., P. Hewitt, and L. Mutch. 1985. Perusing the literature: Comparison of MEDLINE searching with a perinatal trials database. *Controlled Clinical Trials* 6(4):306-317.

Dickersin, K., R. Scherer, and C. Lefebvre. 1994. Identifying relevant studies for systematic reviews. *BMJ* 309(6964):1286-1291.

Dickersin, K., E. Manheimer, S. Wieland, K. A. Robinson, C. Lefebvre, S. McDonald, and the CENTRAL Development Group. 2002. Development of the Cochrane Collaboration's CENTRAL register of controlled clinical trials. *Evaluation and the Health Professions* 25:38-64.

Early Breast Cancer Trialists' Collaborative Group. 1988. Effects of adjuvant tamoxifen and of cytotoxic therapy on mortality in early breast cancer: An overview of 61 randomised trials among 28 896 women. *New England Journal of Medicine* 319:1681-1692.

Easterbrook, P. J., J. A. Berlin, R. Gopalan, and D. R. Matthews. 1991. Publication bias in clinical research. *Lancet* 337:867-872.

Ebrahim, S., and M. Clarke. 2007. STROBE: New standards for reporting observational epidemiology, a chance to improve. *International Journal of Epidemiology* 36(5):945-948.

ECRI. 2006a (unpublished). *2006 ECRI price list*. ECRI Health Technology Assessment Information Service.

———. 2006b. *About ECRI* http://www.ecri.org/About_ECRI/About_ECRI.aspx (accessed January 31, 2007).

Eddy, D. M. 2007. Linking electronic medical records to large-scale simulation models: Can we put rapid learning on turbo? *Health Affairs* 26(2):w125-w136.

Editors. 2005. Reviews: Making sense of an often tangled skein of evidence. *Annals of Internal Medicine* 142(12 Part 1):1019-1020.

Egger, M., T. Zellweger-Zähner, M. Schneider, C. Junker, C. Lengeler, and G. Antes. 1997. Language bias in randomised controlled trials published in English and German. *Lancet* 350(9074):326-329.

Egger, M., G. Davie Smith, and K. O'Rourke. 2001. Rationale, potentials, and promise of systematic reviews. In *Systematic Reviews in Health Care: Meta-Analysis in Context.* Edited by Egger, M. London, UK: BMJ Publishing Group. Pp. 3-19.

Egger, M., P. Juni, C. Bartlett, F. Holenstein, and J. Sterne. 2003. How important are comprehensive literature searches and the assessment of trial quality in systematic reviews? *Health Technology Assessment* 7(1):76.

EPC Coordinating Center. 2005. *Evidence-based practice centers partner's guide* http://www.ahrq.gov/clinic/epcpartner/epcpartner.pdf (accessed January 25, 2007).

Francis, J., and J. B. Perlin. 2006. Improving performance through knowledge translation in the Veterans Health Administration. *Journal of Continuing Education in the Health Professions* 26(1):63-71.

Garfield, E. 2006. The history and meaning of the journal impact factor. *JAMA* 295(1): 90-93.

Glass, G. V. 1976. Primary, secondary and meta-analysis. *Educational Researcher* 5(10):3-8.

Glass, G. V., B. McGaw, and M. L. Smith. 1981. *Meta-analysis in social research.* Newbury Park, CA: Sage Publications.

Glasziou, P., and B. Haynes. 2005. The paths from research to improved health outcomes. *ACP Journal Club* 142(2):A8-A10.

Glasziou, P., J. Vandenbroucke, and I. Chalmers. 2004. Assessing the quality of research. *BMJ* 328(7430):39-41.

Glenny, A. M., M. Esposito, P. Coulthard, and H. V. Worthington. 2003. The assessment of systematic reviews in dentistry. *European Journal of Oral Sciences* 111:85-92.

Gluud, L. L. 2006 Bias in clinical intervention research. *American Journal of Epidemiology* 163(6):493-501.

Goldberger, J. 1907. Typhoid bacillus carriers. Edited by Rosenau, M. J., L. L. Lumsden, and J. H. Kastle. Report on the origin and prevalence of typhoid fever in the District of Columbia. *Hygienic Laboratory Bulletin No. 35* 167-174.

Golder, S., H. M. McIntosh, S. Duffy, and J. Glanville. 2006. Developing efficient search strategies to identify reports of adverse effects in Medline and Embase. *Health Information and Libraries Journal* 23(1):3-12.

Gøtzsche, P. C., A. Hrobjartsson, K. Maric, and B. Tendal. 2007. Data extraction errors in meta-analyses that use standardized mean differences. *JAMA* 298(4):430-437.

GRADE Working Group. 2004. Grading quality of evidence and strength of recommendations. *BMJ* 328(7454):1490.

Guyatt, G. H. 1991. Evidence-based medicine. *ACP Journal Club* 114:A-16.

Harris, R. P., M. Helfand, S. H. Woolf, K. N. Lohr, C. D. Mulrow, S. M. Teutsch, and D. Atkins. 2001. Current methods of the U.S. Preventive Services Task Force: A review of the process. *American Journal of Preventive Medicine* 20(3 Suppl):21-35.

Hayden, J. A., P. Cote, and C. Bombardier. 2006. Evaluation of the quality of prognosis studies in systematic reviews. *Annals of Internal Medicine* 144:427-437.

Hayes, Inc. 2007. *Welcome to Hayes* http://hayesinc.com (accessed May 8, 2007).

Haynes, R. B., D. L. Sackett, G. H. Guyatt, and P. Tugwell. 2006. *Clinical epidemiology: How to do clinical practice research.* 3rd ed. Philadelphia, PA: Lipincott Williams & Wilkins.

The Health Industry Forum. 2006. *Comparative effectiveness forum: Key themes.* Washington, DC: The Health Industry Forum.

Hedges, L. V., and I. Olkin. 1985. *Statistical methods for meta-analysis.* Orlando, FL: Academic Press.

Helfand, M. 2005. Using evidence reports: Progress and challenges in evidence-based decision making. *Health Affairs* 24(1):123-127.

Heres, S., J. Davis, K. Maino, E. Jetzinger, W. Kissling, and S. Leucht. 2006. Why olanzapine beats risperidone, risperidone beats quetiapine, and quetiapine beats olanzapine: An exploratory analysis of head-to-head comparison studies of second-generation antipsychotics. *American Journal of Psychiatry* 163(2):185-194.

Higgins, J. T., and S. Green. 2006. *Cochrane handbook for systematic reviews of interventions 4.2.6 [updated September 2006],* The Cochrane Library, Issue 4, 2006. Chichester, UK: John Wiley & Sons, Ltd.

Hopewell, S., M. Clarke, C. Lefebvre, and R. Scherer. 2007a. Handsearching versus electronic searching to identify reports of randomized trials. *Cochrane Database of Systematic Reviews* (2).

Hopewell, S., S. McDonald, M. Clarke, and M. Egger. 2007b. Grey literature in meta-analyses of randomized trials of health care interventions. *Cochrane Database of Systematic Reviews* (2).

Hypertension. 2007. *Instructions to authors* http://hyper.ahajournals.org/misc/ifora.shtml (accessed July 30, 2007).

ICMJE (International Committee of Medical Journal Editors). 2006. *Uniform requirements for manuscripts submitted to biomedical journals* http://www.icmje.org (accessed September 5, 2007).

Ioannidis, J. P., and J. Lau. 2004. Systematic review of medical evidence. *Journal of Law and Policy* 12(2):509-535.

Ioannidis, J. P., J. W. Evans, P. C. Gøtzsche, R. T. O'Neill, D. Altman, K. Schulz, and D. Moher. 2004. Better reporting of harms in randomized trials: An extension of the CONSORT Statement. *Annals of Internal Medicine* 141:781-788.

IOM (Institute of Medicine). 2007. *Learning what works best: The nation's need for evidence on comparative effectiveness in health care* http://www.iom.edu/ebm-effectiveness (accessed April 2007).

Jadad, A. R., and H. J. McQuay. 1996. Meta-analyses to evaluate analgesic interventions: A systematic qualitative review of their methodology. *Journal of Clinical Epidemiology* 49:235-243.

Jadad, A. R., M. Moher, G. P. Browman, L. Booker, C. Sigouin, M. Fuentes, and R. Stevens. 2000. Systematic reviews and meta-analyses on treatment of asthma: Critical evaluation. *BMJ* 320:537-540.

JAMA. 2007. *Instructions for authors* http://jama.ama-assn.org/misc/ifora.dtl (accessed July 12, 2007).

Jones, A. P., T. Remmington, P. R. Williamson, D. Ashby, and R. L. Smyth. 2005. High prevalence but low impact of data extraction and reporting errors were found in Cochrane systematic reviews. *Journal of Clinical Epidemiology* 58:741-742.

Jorgensen, A. W., J. Hilden, and P. Gøtzsche. 2006. Cochrane reviews compared with industry supported meta-analyses and other meta-analyses of the same drugs: Systematic review. *BMJ Online* 333:782-786.

Journal of Clinical Oncology. 2007. *Information for contributers* http://jco.ascopubs.org/misc/ifora.shtml (accessed July 12, 2007).

Journal of the National Cancer Institute. 2007. *Instructions to authors* http://www.oxfordjournals.org/our_journals/jnci/for_authors/index.html (accessed July 30, 2007).

Khan, K. S., and J. Kleijnen. 2001. Stage II conducting the review: Phase 4 selection of studies. In *CRD Report Number 4.* Edited by Khan, K. S., G. ter Riet, H. Glanville, A. J. Sowden, and J. Kleijnen. York, UK: NHS Centre for Reviews and Dissemination, University of York.

Khan, K. S., J. Popay, and J. Kleijnen. 2001a. Stage I planning the review: Phase 2 development of a review protocol. In *CRD Report Number 4*. Edited by Khan, K. S., G. ter Riet, H. Glanville, A. J. Sowden, and J. Kleijnen. York, UK: NHS Centre for Reviews and Dissemination, University of York.

Khan, K. S., G. ter Riet, J. Popay, J. Nixon, and J. Kleijnen. 2001b. Stage II conducting the review: Phase 5 study quality assessment. In *CRD Report Number 4*. Edited by Khan, K. S., G. ter Riet, H. Glanville, A. J. Sowden, and J. Kleijnen. York, UK: NHS Centre for Reviews and Dissemination, University of York.

Kunz, R., G. Vist, and A. D. Oxman. 2007. Randomisation to protect against selection bias in healthcare trials. *Cochrane Database of Systematic Reviews* (2).

Lancet. 2007. *Information for authors* http://www.thelancet.com/authors/lancet/authorinfo/ (accessed July 30, 2007).

Lau, J., E. M. Antman, J. Jimenez-Silva, B. Kupelnick, F. Mosteller, and T. C. Chalmers. 1992. Cumulative meta-analysis of therapeutic trials for myocardial infarction. *New England Journal of Medicine* 327(4):248-254.

Lavis, J., H. Davies, A. Oxman, J. Denis, K. Golden-Biddle, and E. Ferlie. 2005. Towards systematic reviews that inform health care management and policy-making. *Journal of Health Services Research and Policy* 10(Suppl 1):35-48.

Lexchin, J., L. A. Bero, B. Djulbegovic, and O. Clark. 2003. Pharmaceutical industry sponsorship and research outcome and quality: Systematic review. *BMJ* 326:1167-1170.

Light, R. J., and D. B. Pillemer. 1984. *Summing up*. Cambridge, MA: Harvard University Press.

Mallen, C., G. Peat, and P. Croft. 2006. Quality assessment of observational studies is not commonplace in systematic reviews. *Journal of Clinical Epidemiology* 59:765-769.

Medicare Payment Advisory Commission. 2007. Chapter 2: Producing comparative effectiveness information. In *Report to the Congress: Promoting greater efficiency in Medicare* http://www.medpac.gov/documents/Jun07_EntireReport.pdf (accessed June 2007).

Meyers, D., H. Halvorson, and S. Luckhaupt. 2007. *Evidence synthesis number 48. Screening for chlamydial infection: A focused evidence update for the U.S. Preventive Services Task Force*. Gaithersburg, MD: Agency for Healthcare Research and Quality.

Moher, D., D. J. Cook, S. Eastwood, I. Olkin, D. Rennie, D. F. Stroup, and the QUOROM Group. 1999. Improving the quality of reports of meta-analyses of randomized controlled trials: The QUOROM statement. *Lancet* 354:1896-1900.

Moher, D., A. Jones, L. Lepage, and the CONSORT Group. 2001a. Use of the CONSORT Statement and quality of reports of randomized trials. *JAMA* 285(15):1992-1995.

Moher, D., K. F. Schulz, D. Altman, and the CONSORT Group. 2001b. The CONSORT statement: Revised recommendations for improving the quality of reports of parallel-group randomized trials. *JAMA* 285(15):1987-1991.

Moher, D., J. Tetzlaff, A. C. Tricco, M. Sampson, and D. G. Altman. 2007. Epidemiology and reporting characteristics of systematic reviews. *PLoS Medicine* 4(3):447-455.

Montori, V., N. Wilczynski, D. Morgan, and R. B. Haynes, for the Hedges Team. 2003. Systematic reviews: A cross-sectional study of location and citation counts. *BMC Medicine* 1(1):2.

Mulrow, C. 1987. The medical review article: State of the science. *Annals of Internal Medicine* 106:485-488.

Mulrow, C., and K. Lohr. 2001. Proof and policy from medical research evidence. *Journal of Health Politics, Policy and Law* 26(2):249-266.

Mulrow, C. D., D. J. Cook, and F. Davidoff. 1997. Systematic reviews: Critical links in the great chain of evidence. *Annals of Internal Medicine* 126(5):389-391.

Neumann, P. J. 2006. Emerging lessons from the Drug Effectiveness Review Project. *Health Affairs* 25(4):w262-w271.

Neumann, P. J., N. Divi, M. T. Beinfeld, B. S. Levine, P. S. Keenan, E. F. Halpern, and
    G. S. Gazelle. 2005. Medicare's national coverage decisions, 1999-2003: Quality of
    evidence and review times. *Health Affairs* 24(1):243-254.
Neumann, P. J., N. Divi, M. T. Beinfeld, and B. S. Levine. 2007 (unpublished). *Medicare
    National Coverage Decision Database.* Tufts-New England Medical Center. Sponsored
    by the Commonwealth Fund.
New England Journal of Medicine. 2007. *Instructions for submitting a NEW manuscript*
    http://authors.nejm.org/Misc/NewMS.asp (accessed July 12, 2007).
NGC (National Guideline Clearinghouse). 2007. *Search for cardiology* http://www.guideline.
    gov/search/searchresults.aspx?Type=3&txtSearch=cardiology&num=500 (accessed July
    11, 2007).
Norris, S. L., and D. Atkins. 2005. Challenges in using nonrandomized studies in system-
    atic reviews of treatment interventions. *Annals of Internal Medicine* 142(12 Part 2):
    1112-1119.
Obstetrics and Gynecology. 2007. *Instructions for authors* http://www.greenjournal.org/misc/
    authors.pdf (accessed July 12, 2007).
Oxman, A. D., and G. H. Guyatt. 1988. Guidelines for reading literature reviews. *Canadian
    Medical Association Journal* 138:697-703.
Oxman, A. D., H. J. Schünemann, and A. Fretheim. 2006. Improving the use of research evi-
    dence in guideline development: 7. Deciding what evidence to include. *Health Research
    Policy and Systems* 4(19).
Pearson, K. 1904. Report on certain enteric fever inoculation statistics. *BMJ* 3:1243-1246.
Pediatrics. 2007. *Instructions for authors* http://mc.manuscriptcentral.com/societyimages/
    pediatrics/2004_author_instructions.pdf (accessed July 12, 2007).
Peppercorn, J., E. Blood, E. Winer, and A. Partridge. 2007. Association between pharmaceutical
    involvement and outcomes in breast cancer clinical trials. *Cancer* 109(7):1239-1246.
Perlin, J. B., and J. Kupersmith. 2007. Information technology and the inferential gap. *Health
    Affairs* 26(2):w192-w194.
Poolman, R., P. Struijs, R. Krips, I. Sierevelt, K. Lutz, and M. Bhandari. 2006. Does a "Level I
    Evidence" rating imply high quality of reporting in orthopaedic randomised controlled
    trials? *BMC Medical Research Methodology* 6(1):44.
Pratt, J. G., J. B. Rhine, B. M. Smith, C. E. Stuart, and J. A. Greenwood. 1940. *Extra-sensory
    perception after sixty years: A critical appraisal of the research in extra-sensory percep-
    tion.* New York: Henry Holt.
Radiology. 2007. *Publication information for authors* http://www.rsna.org/publications/rad/
    pdf/pia.pdf (accessed July 11, 2007).
Rayleigh, L. 1884. Address by the Rt. Hon. Lord Rayleigh. In *Report of the fifty-fourth
    meeting of the British Association for the Advancement of Science.* Edited by Murray,
    J. Montreal.
Reviews in Clinical Gerontology. 2007. *Instructions for contributors* http://assets.cambridge.
    org/RCG/RCG_ifc.pdf (accessed July 30, 2007).
Richardson, W. S., M. C. Wilson, J. Nishikawa, and R. S. A. Hayward. 1995. The well-built
    clinical question: A key to evidence-based decisions [editorial]. *ACP Journal Club* 123:
    A12-A13.
Rietveld, R. P., H. C. P. M. van Weert, G. ter Riet, and P. J. E. Bindels. 2003. Diagnostic
    impact of signs and symptoms in acute infectious conjunctivitis: Systematic literature
    search. *BMJ* 327(7418):789.
Rosenthal, R. 1978. Combining results of independent studies. *Psychological Bulletin* 85:
    185-193.
Santaguida, P., M. Helfand, and P. Raina. 2005. Challenges in systematic reviews that evaluate
    drug efficacy or effectiveness. *Annals of Internal Medicine* 142(12 Part 2):1066-1072.

Scherer, R. W., P. Langenberg, and E. von Elm. 2007. Full publication of results initially presented in abstracts. *Cochrane Database of Systematic Reviews* (2).

Scholes, D., A. Stergachis, F. E. Heidrich, H. Andrilla, K. K. Holmes, and W. E. Stamm. 1996. Prevention of pelvic inflammatory disease by screening for cervical chlamydial infection. *New England Journal of Medicine* 334(21):1362-1366.

Schünemann, H., D. Best, G. Vist, and A. D. Oxman. 2003. Letters, numbers, symbols and words: How to communicate grades of evidence and recommendations. *Canadian Medical Association Journal* 169(7):677-680.

Schünemann, H., A. Oxman, and A. Fretheim. 2006. Improving the use of research evidence in guideline development: 6. Determining which outcomes are important. *Health Research Policy and Systems* 4(1):18.

Shea, B., D. Moher, I. Graham, B. A. Pham, and P. Tugwell. 2002. A comparison of the quality of Cochrane reviews and systematic reviews published in paper-based journals. *Evaluation and the Health Professions* 25:116-129.

Shekelle, P. G., E. Ortiz, S. Rhodes, S. C. Morton, M. P. Eccles, J. M. Grimshaw, and S. H. Woolf. 2001. Validity of the Agency for Healthcare Research and Quality Clinical Practice Guidelines: How quickly do guidelines become outdated? *JAMA* 286:1461-1467.

Shojania, K. G., M. Sampson, M. T. Ansari, J. Ji, S. Doucette, and D. Moher. 2007. How quickly do systematic reviews go out of date? A survival analysis. *Annals of Internal Medicine* 147:224-233.

Sinclair, J., and M. Bracken. 1992. *Effective care of the newborn infant.* New York: Oxford University Press.

Slutsky, J. 2007. *Approaches to priority setting: Identifying topics and selection. Submitted Responses to the HECS Committee Meeting, January 25, 2007.* Washington, DC.

Song, F., A. J. Eastwood, S. Gilbody, L. Duley, and A. J. Sutton. 2000. Publication and related biases. *Health Technology Assessment* 4(10).

Spine. 2007. *Instructions for authors* http://edmgr.ovid.com/spine/accounts/ifauth.htm (accessed July 12, 2007).

Steinberg, E. P., and B. R. Luce. 2005. Evidence based? Caveat emptor! *Health Affairs* 24(1):80-92.

Stewart, W. F., N. R. Shah, M. J. Selna, R. A. Paulus, and J. M. Walker. 2007. Bridging the inferential gap: The electronic health record and clinical evidence. *Health Affairs* 26(2): w181-w191.

Stroup, D. F., J. A. Berlin, S. C. Morton, I. Olkin, G. D. Williamson, D. Rennie, D. Moher, B. J. Becker, T. A. Sipe, and S. B. Thacker for the Meta-analysis Of Observational Studies in Epidemiology (MOOSE) Group. 2000. Meta-analysis of observational studies in epidemiology: A proposal for reporting. *JAMA* 283(15):2008-2012.

Sutton, A. J., K. R. Abrams, D. R. Jones, T. A. Sheldon, and F. Song. 2000. *Methods for meta-analysis in medical research.* London, UK: John Wiley.

Tatsioni, A., D. A. Zarin, N. Aronson, D. J. Samson, C. R. Flamm, C. Schmid, and J. Lau. 2005. Challenges in systematic reviews of diagnostic technologies. *Annals of Internal Medicine* 142(12 Part 2):1048-1055.

Treadwell, J. R., S. J. Tregear, J. T. Reston, and C. M. Turkelson. 2006. A system for rating the stability and strength of medical evidence. *BMC Medical Research Methodology [electronic resource]* 6:52.

Tunis, S. 2006. *Improving evidence for health care decisions. Presentation to IOM staff, April 28, 2006.* Washington, DC.

USPSTF (U.S. Preventive Services Task Force). 2007. *U.S. Preventive Services Task Force ratings* http://www.ahrq.gov/clinic/uspstf07/ratingsv2.htm (accessed July 10, 2007).

von Elm, E., D. G. Altman, M. Egger, S. J. Pocock, P. C. Gøtzsche, J. P. Vandenbroucke, and the Strobe Initiative. 2007. The Strengthening the Reporting of Observational Studies in Epidemiology (STROBE) Statement: Guidelines for reporting observational studies. *Annals of Internal Medicine* 147(8):573-577.

West, S., V. King, T. Carey, K. Lohr, N. McCoy, S. Sutton, and L. Lux. 2002. *Systems to rate the strength of scientific evidence. Evidence Report/Technology Assessment No. 47. (Prepared by the Research Triangle Institute-University of North Carolina Evidence-based Practice Center under Contract No. 290-97-0011.) AHRQ Publication No. 02-E016.* Rockville, MD: Agency for Healthcare Research and Quality.

Whiting, P., A. W. Rutjes, J. Dinnes, J. B. Reitsma, P. M. Bossuyt, and J. Kleijnen. 2005. A systematic review finds that diagnostic reviews fail to incorporate quality despite available tools. *Journal of Clinical Epidemiology* 58:1-12.

Wieland, S., and K. Dickersin. 2005. Selective exposure reporting and Medline indexing limited the search sensitivity for observational studies of the adverse effects of oral contraceptives. *Journal of Clinical Epidemiology* 58(6):560-567.

Wilczynski, N. L., D. Morgan, R. B. Haynes, and the Hedges Team. 2005. An overview of the design and methods for retrieving high-quality studies for clinical care. *BMC Medical Informatics and Decision Making* 5(20).

Wilensky, G. R. 2006. Developing a center for comparative effectiveness information. *Health Affairs* w572.

World Health Organization. 2007. *International clinical trials registry platform* http://www. who.int/ictrp/en/ (accessed August 9, 2007).

Yusuf, S., R. Peto, J. Lewis, R. Collins, and P. Sleight. 1985. Beta blockade during and after myocardial infarction: An overview of the randomized trials. *Progress in Cardiovascular Diseases* 27(5):335-371.

5

Developing Trusted Clinical Practice Guidelines

Abstract: This chapter reviews the current landscape of clinical practice guideline development in the United States, presents the committee recommendations for creating trusted clinical practice guidelines, and describes key challenges in promoting the development and adoption of high-quality guidelines under the aegis of a proposed national clinical effectiveness assessment program ("the Program"). Under the status quo, the processes underlying guideline development are often vulnerable to bias and conflict of interest. Overall, the quality of clinical practice guidelines is often poor. The committee recommends that the Program establish standards for guideline development but also promote voluntary adoption of Program standards by guideline developers. The standards must address the composition of guidelines panels to ensure that guidelines are created by a diversity and balance of competing interests with minimal bias. The standards should also promote objectivity, transparency, and efficiency in guideline development and clear, standardized reporting of clinical recommendations. Groups developing clinical practice guidelines should document their adherence to Program standards and make this documentation publicly available. Individuals and organizations that utilize guideline information would then be in a better position to assess guideline quality and utilize only those guidelines that meet the Program's standards.

The development of clinical practice guidelines for use by practitioners, payers, patients, and others is a key strategy in promoting the use of highly effective clinical services. When they are used, rigorously developed guidelines have the potential to reduce undesirable practice variation, reduce the use of services that are of minimal or questionable value, increase the utilization of services that are effective but underused, and target services to those populations most likely to benefit (Grimshaw and Russell, 1993).

Underlying the effort to produce evidence-based guidelines is a pressing need for trusted information on clinical effectiveness. As described earlier, in recent years there has been a substantial increase in the number of treatment alternatives available to providers and patients, as well as in the volume of studies describing the effectiveness (or ineffectiveness) of those options. This body of evidence has become complex and difficult to manage for most providers. As a result, guidelines have become a key tool for summarizing the available literature and placing it in a format accessible to physicians (Druss and Marcus, 2005).

This chapter has three principal objectives: (1) to review the current landscape of clinical practice guideline development in the United States, (2) to present the committee's recommendations for creating trusted clinical practice guidelines, and (3) to highlight key challenges in promoting the development and adoption of high-quality guidelines under the aegis of a proposed national clinical effectiveness assessment program ("the Program").

BACKGROUND

Clinical practice guidelines attempt to define practices that meet the needs of most patients under most circumstances. They do not attempt to supplant the independent judgment of clinicians in responding to particular clinical situations. Ideally, the specific clinical recommendations that are contained within practice guidelines have been systematically developed by panels of experts who have access to the available evidence, an understanding of the clinical problem and the relevant research methods, and sufficient time to absorb the information and make considered judgments (GRADE Working Group, 2004). These panels are expected to be objective and to produce recommendations that are unbiased, up-to-date, and free from conflict of interest.

Groups that measure provider performance frequently use adherence to clinical practice guidelines as a basis upon which to evaluate the quality of care, and many payers are now moving toward the use of pay-for-performance strategies that establish differential payments on the basis of adherence to quality measures. In addition to performance-based payment, with the increased use of health information technology and direct decision support at the point of care, guidelines are likely to become increasingly influential in clinical practice (O'Malley et al., 2007).

Perhaps the earliest guidelines produced in the United States were the American Academy of Pediatrics' Redbook of Infectious Diseases, published in the 1930s (American Academy of Pediatrics, 2007). The groups that were among the first to use systematic reviews to support clinical recommendations were the Canadian Task Force on the Periodic Health Examination and the U.S. Preventive Services Task Force (USPSTF) (Fielding and Briss, 2006). The Canadian task force was established in 1976 to make recommendations about the inclusion of preventive services in the periodic health examination; the USPSTF was established in 1984 and also provided prevention-related recommendations for health professionals (Woolf and Atkins, 2001). The American College of Physicians began to publish explicit recommendations based on systematic reviews in 1981 (Eddy, 2005).

In 1989, Congress established the Agency for Health Care Policy and Research (AHCPR) and tasked it with developing clinical practice guidelines, among its other responsibilities. The Institute of Medicine (IOM) noted that this effort was part of a cultural shift: a move away from an unexamined reliance on professional judgment and toward more structured support and accountability for these judgments (1990). Before the move toward evidence-based practice, medical textbooks and articles were filled with thousands of statements and care recommendations that were based solely on the belief of the author or at best a consensus of experts (Eddy, 2005). Evidence-based guidelines initiatives aim to base recommendations on empirical evidence.

Relationship to Systematic Reviews

Clinical guidelines go beyond systematic reviews by recommending what should and should not be done in specific clinical circumstances. Although systematic reviews produce findings about clinical effectiveness, transforming that evidence into specific care recommendations is often challenging. Given the gaps in information that frequently exist and the variable quality of the information that is available, a key component of guideline development is the establishment of a link between the strength of the clinical recommendation and the quality of the underlying evidence.

Guyatt and colleagues (2006a) argue that one of the first criteria of an effective guideline development process is having two separate grading systems: one for the quality of the evidence and another for the recommendations themselves. The quality of evidence grade reflects the level of confidence that, if the recommendation is followed, the anticipated outcomes will occur. The strength of the recommendation takes into account the balance of the benefits and the harms that are associated with the intervention and the guideline authors' views about the importance of adhering to the recommendation.

Resource Requirements

Guideline production requires a significant commitment by professional societies and others who perform the work, especially if they conduct high-quality systematic reviews themselves. Locating and analyzing all of the available evidence requires substantial skills, resources, and time, and professional groups often lack what is needed to do a credible job (Woolf et al., 1999). The resource demands of conducting a rigorous systematic review often leads guideline developers to revert to short-cuts or processes centered on expert opinion (Browman, 2001). Moreover, a substantial investment in evidence gathering does not guarantee a good return on evidence available to address a question (Ricci et al., 2006). In fact, guideline developers often must reckon with research that is not sufficiently rigorous, yields conflicting results, or does not exist (Cook and Giacomini, 1999). This also contributes to pressures to rely more heavily on professional opinion.

Guideline Developers[1]

As described in Chapter 2, many groups produce clinical practice guidelines and recommendations. The National Guideline Clearinghouse (NGC) currently includes guidelines from approximately 360 organizations (NGC, 2007c). Medical professional societies are the most common sponsors of guidelines. In addition, patient advocacy groups, payers, government agencies, and others in the United States may conduct systematic reviews and develop clinical recommendations. Organizations in other countries also produce guidelines that are available in the United States, including the National Institute for Health and Clinical Excellence (NICE), the Scottish Intercollegiate Guidelines Network (SIGN), and organizations in Australia and Canada.

In the United States, the NGC provides free access to guidelines produced across a range of clinical areas. The NGC included approximately 650 guidelines in 1999 (O'Connor, 2005) and has grown to nearly 2,200 guidelines today (NGC, 2007b). The website now receives an estimated 1.3 million visits per month.[2] For a guideline to be included on the website, guideline producers are required to demonstrate that they performed a systematic literature search and that they developed, reviewed, or revised the guideline within the last five years (NGC, 2007a). By meeting NGC standards and being admitted to the website, guideline developers are able to improve the dissemination of their products.

---

[1]See Chapter 2 for background on organizations that develop or use clinical practice guidelines.

[2]Personal communication, J. Slutsky, Agency for Healthcare Research and Quality, September 4, 2007.

The USPSTF, having been in existence for over 20 years, serves as a model of recommendation development in the United States, especially because of its adherence to detailed methodologies and the restrictions it places on conflicts of interest. Clinicians, health plans, and payers have come to rely on the regular reports from the task force to update their practice, payment, or coverage policies regarding clinical preventive services.

CURRENT LANDSCAPE

Quality of Guidelines

The IOM Committee on Clinical Practice Guidelines defined high-quality guidelines as having a number of attributes, including validity, reliability, reproducibility, clinical applicability and flexibility, clarity, development through a multidisciplinary process, scheduled reviews, and documentation (IOM, 1992). Over time there have been noted improvements in the capacities of some clinical and professional organizations to develop robust, evidence-based guidelines (Jackson and Feder, 1998). Nevertheless, the overall quality of clinical practice guidelines is highly variable, and in fact, the quality is often very poor (Shaneyfelt et al., 1999). Shaneyfelt and colleagues (1999) assessed the quality of 279 guidelines produced over the period of 1985 to 1997 and assessed their quality against a set of 25 standards. The investigators found that the mean number of quality standards satisfied over that period was 11 (43 percent). For example, less than 10 percent of the guidelines described formal methods of combining scientific evidence and expert opinion. The investigators also evaluated the guidelines in accordance to their specification of purpose (75 percent compliance), definition of the patient population involved (46 percent), pertinent health outcomes (40 percent), method of external review (32 percent), and whether an expiration date or scheduled update was included (11 percent). Overall, the investigation found significant improvement over time, but each guideline still only met 50 percent of the standards, on average, in 1997 (Shaneyfelt et al., 1999). For some, this variability in guideline quality called for greater transparency in guideline reporting and more rigorous peer review (Cook and Giacomini, 1999).

An evaluation of 86 guidelines developed in 11 countries (which did not include the United States) concluded that the guidelines produced by government-funded agencies and established guideline development programs were of higher quality than guidelines produced by specialty societies (Burgers, 2003). This finding was consistent with the conclusions of Grilli and colleagues (2000), and also with Hasenfeld and Shekelle (2003), who found that the 17 guidelines produced by the AHCPR from 1990 to 1996 were of a substantially higher quality than those subsequently produced by other groups. The authors postulated that the higher-quality scores of guidelines developed by government agencies reflect the fact that the production of high-quality guidelines requires substantial and sufficient resources and that government agencies have more resources available to do the work.

Smaller professional organizations often lack the internal resources, including staff capacity and expertise, required to produce guidelines. This is especially true when the organization produces both the systematic reviews and the guideline recommendations, two tasks requiring different skill sets. Even larger professional organizations can face resource constraints in this area. Some have suggested that, given these resource constraints, government is in the best position to produce clinical practice guidelines (Burgers, 2003; Hasenfeld and Shekelle, 2003).

Many of the criticisms directed at the U.S. system of guideline production in 1990 still apply today (IOM, 1990). These criticisms focused on conflicting clinical recommendations; failure to address certain topics; and incomplete public disclosure of the evidence surveyed, methods used, composition of the panel, and conflicts of interest. In addition, it remains true that, aside from the role that AHRQ plays in populating the NGC website, no independent entity exists in the United States to certify guideline quality or to develop national standards regulating the content or methods of guideline developers. The 1990 IOM report *Clinical Practice Guidelines: Directions for a New Program* sought to encourage more standardization and consistency in guideline development, and although the quality of clinical practice guidelines has generally improved since then, substantial inconsistencies in the methodologies and reporting language used still exist (Guyatt et al., 2006b; Shiffman et al., 2003).

Quality of Information

The translation of systematic reviews into practice recommendations is not straightforward. The same information can be interpreted in different ways by different panelists, resulting in the provision of different guidance (Burgers and van Everdingen, 2004). Often, even when there is substantial consensus about what the scientific evidence says, there are disagreements about what the evidence means for clinical practice. Conclusions about clinical effectiveness can vary widely as a result of conflicting viewpoints, such as which outcomes are the most important and which course of action is appropriate given that the evidence is imperfect (Atkins et al., 2005b). This section highlights strategies that guideline developers have used to improve the reliability and trustworthiness of the information that they provide. It also examines methodological approaches, and how groups have sought to ensure objectivity in their procedures. Finally, this section examines assessments of the overall quality of the recommendations currently being made.

Methodological Rigor

Although there have been recent efforts to standardize approaches to guideline development, it is not yet possible to say that guideline development is based on a scientifically validated process. The key challenges stem from the fact that guideline development frequently forces organizations to go beyond what is known from a scientific point of view to make practical recommendations for use in everyday practice. Two examples of such challenges are the approaches to limitations in the evidence base and subjective assessments of the net benefit.

Limitations of the evidence base The evidence base that supports clinical practice guidelines is often quite limited and guideline developers must often wrestle with what to do when "the irresistible force of the need to offer clinical advice meets with the immovable object of flawed evidence" (Ricci et al., 2006, p. 229). They must consider the best way to address the trade-off between rigor and pragmatism (Browman, 2001), and between adherence to evidence and broader clinical utility (Perlin and Kupersmith, 2007; Stewart et al., 2007). As a result, a consensus of expert opinion among clinical and methodologist panelists often fills in the gaps between areas supported by scientific evidence.

In making their treatment decisions, practicing clinicians might want to place less reliance on guidelines that are based primarily on expert opinion rather than empirical evidence. Often, however, it is not clear which parts of guidelines are evidence-based, and which are not. Many times, when groups incorporate expert opinion, they do not do so in a standardized way (Thomson et al., 1998). The methods for incorporating opinion into guidelines is less well-developed than the methods for incorporating research results and often they are not made explicit. Disclosing the role of expert opinion is especially important when the data are sparse (Cook and Giacomini, 1999).

When combining a review of research data with practice recommendations, guidelines often do not identify an explicit search strategy used, do not have defined inclusion criteria for selecting eligible studies, and do not assess the findings against consistent methodological standards (Miller and Petrie, 2000). Guidelines such as these often reflect a subjective assessment of the consistency, clinical relevance, and external validity of the available evidence (Ricci et al., 2006).

Subjective assessments of net benefit   The development of clinical recommendations should involve a summary of the harms and benefits of a particular service or intervention. The strength of the recommendation reflects this assessment. Table 5-1 illustrates how the USPSTF addresses net benefit in its strength of recommendation categories.

Although some bodies of evidence show a high degree of benefit and few harms, in many cases the benefit and harm seem to be more closely balanced and it is much more difficult to justify a strong recommendation. In situations in which the evidence is of poor quality, it may be difficult to come to an agreement about the balance between the benefits and harms (Atkins et al., 2005a). However, even when the data and the evidence are solid, value judgments come into play when making these assessments (Woolf et al., 1999).

Rendering judgments about evidence and the subsequent development of appropriate recommendations are complex and the use of some sub-

TABLE 5-1 USPSTF Strength of Recommendations

Grade	Definition	Suggestions for Practice
A	The USPSTF recommends the service. There is high certainty that the net benefit is substantial.	Offer or provide this service.
B	The USPSTF recommends the service. There is high certainty that the net benefit is moderate or there is moderate certainty that the net benefit is moderate to substantial.	Offer or provide this service.
C	The USPSTF recommends against routinely providing the service. There may be considerations that support providing the service in an individual patient. There is at least moderate certainty that the net benefit is small.	Offer or provide this service only if other considerations support the offering or providing the service in an individual patient.
D	The USPSTF recommends against the service. There is moderate or high certainty that the service has no net benefit or that the harms outweigh the benefits.	Discourage the use of this service.
I	The USPSTF concludes that the current evidence is insufficient to assess the balance of benefits and harms of the service. Evidence is lacking, of poor quality, or conflicting, and the balance of benefits and harms cannot be determined.	Read the clinical considerations section of USPSTF Recommendation Statement. If the service is offered, patients should understand the uncertainty about the balance of benefits and harms.

SOURCE: AHRQ (2007).

jectivity in the process is unavoidable (Atkins et al., 2005a). Inconsistent recommendations from different practice guideline development committees often reflect differences in values and tolerances for potential harm. People may perceive the importance of a specific health outcome differently and thus may differ on the point at which the likely benefits of a treatment outweigh the likely harms (IOM, 1990). Guyatt and colleagues (2006a) have indicated that when value or preference judgments are particularly important to the recommendation, guideline development panels should describe the key values attached to these outcomes, and how they influenced the content or strength of the recommendation.

Guideline development panels often do not include patients or consumers as members, and they may not seek patient input when weighing particular health states (Guyatt et al., 2006a). However, some patient and consumer advocacy groups are taking a more prominent role in the evidence-based health care field, and the concept of shared decision making has begun to take hold. The use of decision aids is bringing objective information about benefits and harms directly to patients so that they and their physicians can make informed and appropriate decisions (Weinstein et al., 2007). Shared decision making is often the best approach for elective procedures, for example, in deciding whether an arthritic knee hurts enough to justify the risks of knee replacement.

Addressing Bias

Patients, clinicians, payers, purchasers, and many others rely on having clinical recommendations that are produced in an objective manner. Groups making clinical recommendations have attempted to ensure objectivity in a variety of ways. The following sections examine in detail measures that promote the formation of panels with a balanced composition of members and freedom from conflict of interest.

Panel composition To protect against a bias in perspective, it is important that guideline development panels include individuals from a range of relevant professional groups. Panels that are composed of members from a single specialty are likely to reach conclusions different from those of panels with multispecialty representation, even when both panels are presented with the same set of evidence (Shekelle et al., 1999). Kahan and colleagues (1996) examined six surgical procedures and found that between 10 and 42 percent of all cases that were deemed appropriate by specialists who performed the procedure were deemed less than appropriate by primary care providers. Murphy and colleagues (1998) found that members of a specialty are more likely to advocate the use of techniques that involve their specialty. Possible explanations for these systematic differences in judgment include superior knowledge, economic self-interest, and inadvertent cognitive bias (Kahan et al., 1996).

To address some of the problems noted, many researchers and others have encouraged the use of balanced, multidisciplinary panels that include representatives from different clinical specialties as well as methodologists and patients. For example, the RAND Corporation-University of California at Los Angeles appropriateness method employs a nine-member multidisciplinary panel to assess the appropriateness of specific interventions for specific indications. These panels include specialists who perform the procedure in question, specialists who do not perform the procedure but have practices in related areas (e.g., noninvasive cardiologists for a coronary arteriography panel), and primary care providers (e.g., internists).

Shekelle and colleagues (1999) have argued that guideline development panels with multidisciplinary representation may produce more reliable results because such a structure can balance the biases of the various individuals on the panel. The IOM Committee to Advise the Public Health Service on Clinical Practice Guidelines found that multidisciplinary participation (1) increases the probability that all relevant scientific evidence will be located and critically evaluated, (2) increases the chances that the committee will address practical problems relating to application of the guidelines, and (3) helps build support among the groups for whom the guideline is intended (IOM, 1990).

However, the specific make-up of guideline development panels often remains unaffected by these findings. Grilli and colleagues (2000) examined the guidelines produced by specialty societies and found that only 28 percent mentioned the inclusion of a panelist of a different specialty. Others most often invited to participate included epidemiologists or methodologists, primary care physicians, health administrators, and patients or consumer representatives (Grilli et al., 2000). Another study found that only 26 percent of the guidelines examined provided a description of the participants included in the guideline development process along with their areas of expertise (Shaneyfelt et al., 1999).

Conflicts of interest[3]   Actual and perceived conflicts of interest are a major source of concern for stakeholders seeking objective assessments about clinical effectiveness. These conflicts can occur when decision makers—including individual clinicians and clinicians serving on guideline development panels—have a personal stake in the outcome of the decision, such

---

[3] A recently formed IOM Committee on Conflict of Interest in Medical Research, Education, and Practice is studying conflicts of interest in the conduct of medical research, development of practice guidelines, and patient care. A final report is expected in 2009.

as a potential financial gain or the loss of intellectual standing (i.e., reputation). In the past several years, these types of conflicts of interest among decision makers have come under increasing scrutiny. Because the interpretation of scientific evidence and its translation into clinical decisions often involve the use of a substantial amount of judgment, conflicts of interest add to concerns that bias may be injected into the process.

One recent survey of physicians found that 94 percent have some type of relationship with the pharmaceutical industry (Campbell et al., 2007). More than one-third reported that they had received reimbursement for costs associated with professional meetings or continuing medical education; and 28 percent reported that they had received payments for consulting, lecturing, or enrolling patients in clinical trials. For many, there is a persistent concern that these relationships have an undue impact on treatment decisions, creating risks for individual patients, and undermining the integrity of the medical profession (Tonelli, 2007). For example, a recent analysis conducted by the *New York Times* concluded that from 1997 through 2005, Minnesota physicians who received the most money from makers of atypical antipsychotic drugs were more likely to prescribe the drugs to children (Harris et al., 2007). On average, Minnesota psychiatrists who received at least $5,000 from the makers of atypical antipsychotic drugs from 2000 to 2005 wrote three times as many atypical prescriptions for children as psychiatrists who received less or no money, according to the authors.

In addition, investigators' public positions on drug safety can be associated with their financial relationships with pharmaceutical manufacturers. For example, investigators who supported the use of calcium-channel antagonists were significantly more likely to have a financial relationship with manufacturers, as compared to those who took a neutral or critical position (90, 60, and 37 percent respectively) (Stelfox, 1998).

Conflict of interest is a problem for guideline developers as well. In a survey of clinical practice guideline authors, 59 percent indicated that they had a relationship with companies whose products were included in the guideline that they authored (Choudhry et al., 2002). Aside from equity interest in the companies being evaluated, other types of conflicts include receipt of royalties, speakers fees, consulting fees, and research funding for unrelated products, in addition to various types of intellectual conflicts of interest.

The public and Congress have become concerned about perceptions of conflict of interest at both the U.S. Food and Drug Administration (FDA) and the National Institutes of Health (NIH). Both agencies have recently promulgated new guidelines that limit the amount of money that external advisory panel members can receive from companies whose products or services may be a focus of their review. In addition, several medical schools have placed restrictions on the access that pharmaceutical sales representatives can have to their students.

Public disclosure is a highly touted remedy for the biases that may be inherent in conflicted relationships (Choudhry et al., 2002; Stelfox, 1998). For example, Boyd and Bero (2006) recommend the use of specific, detailed, and structured—rather than open-ended—forms to solicit as much information as possible about the nature and extent of the conflict. They recommend the disclosure of all financial ties publicly. In cases in which the conflicts appear to be intractable, they recommend that panelists recuse themselves from decisions.

However, Jerome Kassirer (2007), former editor-in-chief of the *New England Journal of Medicine*, argues that transparency measures are insufficient and may actually be harmful because they divert attention away from the more difficult problem, which is protecting the integrity of medical information. Kassirer maintains that there should be a lower threshold of concern about financial conflicts and that although small numbers of conflicted individuals should be allowed to participate in review panels, they should not be given an opportunity to vote on recommendations pertaining to their financial interests. The challenge, however, is that so many health professionals have conflicts, including those with the greatest expertise.

Professional societies are subject to internal and external pressures to support certain practices. Societies may depend on commercial relationships for operating and educational funds. Moreover, specialty societies engaged in market-based competition with each other may publish guidelines that are intended to help them gain ownership of the specific procedures or treatments (Woolf et al., 1999). In addition, individual guideline developers may have a substantial economic or professional stake in the intervention being considered. This has the potential to produce recommendations that ignore or minimize harms or that overestimate the benefit of an intervention (Schwartz, 1984).

Pluralistic Approach to Guideline Development

The current approach to developing clinical recommendations in the United States is highly decentralized. Many different organizations participate in the process, which allows broad participation by private stakeholders. In addition, rather than having government serve as the primary financier of guideline development, the current system enables the costs to be spread out among multiple parties.

Although public sector groups that develop guidelines are less central to the guideline development process than they once were, they still play a significant role. The USPSTF continues to produce recommendations for preventive services that are widely considered to be the "gold standard" for the process of guideline development (Guirguis-Blake et al., 2007). The task force maintains a rigorous process for contracting with evidence-based practice centers (EPCs) to produce systematic reviews and developing practice recommendations; it sets a high standard for other organizations.

The NIH also convenes expert panels to develop clinical recommendations. For example, the National Heart, Lung, and Blood Institute (NHLBI) launched the National Cholesterol Education Program in November 1985 and now sponsors a number of panels that produce guidelines in that area. The NIH Consensus Development Conferences also seek to inform clinical practice, and now contracts with EPCs for systematic reviews of the evidence, although they do not produce practice guidelines.

Multiple Conflicting Guidelines

One of the challenges inherent in having such a decentralized, pluralistic process is that often multiple groups produce guidelines in the same clinical topic area. These guidelines may duplicate previous work or produce contradictory findings that may remain unresolved (Woolf et al., 1999). Box 5-1 illustrates a case in which two guideline development panels reviewed largely the same bodies of evidence and reached different conclusions about appropriate clinical practice.

The magnitude of this challenge is illustrated by the preponderance of guidelines related to hypertension and stroke. The NGC, for example,

---

BOX 5-1
Conflicting Guidelines for the Treatment of Epilepsy

Separate panels convened in the United States and the United Kingdom looked at the use of new antiepileptic drugs for the treatment of newly diagnosed epilepsy patients. Although both groups supported the efficacy and safety of the new drugs, they diverged on the appropriate management of these cases. The U.S. panel recommended that either the new drugs or the standard drugs be used (depending on the characteristics of the patient), whereas the U.K. panel was more restrictive, recommending that the new drugs be used only in more narrow circumstances (e.g., cases where the older drug is contraindicated). These discrepancies may be partially explained by the limited amount of information available on the new drugs and the different factors considered by the reviewers (e.g., the U.K. review considered cost and quality of life, but the U.S. review did not). It is also likely that more subjective judgments play a role in the recommendation process.

SOURCE: Beghi (2004).

includes 471 hypertension guidelines and 276 stroke guidelines (NGC, 2007e,f). Anyone looking to ferret out pertinent information faces a substantial sifting process and challenges in determining which of the guidelines are the most relevant and trustworthy. Although the NGC allows readers to compare the guidelines side by side across a number of dimensions, this feature quickly becomes unwieldy as the number of relevant guidelines increases. In addition, the guidelines differ substantially in the way that they present information, making it difficult for the reader to compare one set of findings directly against another. For example, guidelines employ different rating scales to characterize the quality of the supporting evidence (see below).

Gap Areas

Despite the overabundance of clinical guidance in some topic areas, little guidance exists in other important areas. The following examples illustrate how gaps in guideline production may occur:

- Some commonly used treatments may not have been examined in systematic reviews, primarily because of a lack of agreement on which professional society "owns" the condition (e.g., treatments for prostate cancer, which may be "owned" by the American Urological Association, the American Society of Clinical Oncology, or the American Society for Therapeutic Radiology and Oncology).
- Researchers may avoid doing reviews of treatments for rare and "orphan" diseases either because the evidence is weak, because no entity is identified as being responsible for developing a guideline, or because there is inadequate financial support to conduct the work.
- Some professional societies may not produce guidelines at all because they do not view it as a part of their mission, or they may release clinical position statements that have very little evidentiary basis.
- Given the speed at which medicine is changing, guideline production by professional societies may fall behind what is known about new knowledge and technology.

Efforts to Improve Guidelines

Consensus Building

Recognizing that in some clinical areas multiple organizations may seek to develop guidelines, some groups have developed collaborative activities that promote consensus in clinical practice guidelines. For example, the

American College of Cardiology (ACC) and the American Heart Association (AHA) have jointly produced clinical practice guidelines since the 1980s. Because their guidelines are intended for use by a broad range of health providers, the ACC/AHA writing committees often include representatives of other organizations, including other groups specializing in the cardiovascular field, such as the American College of Chest Physicians, and other specialties such as the American Academy of Family Practice and the American College of Physicians. In seeking to develop consensus guidelines, the NHLBI's National Cholesterol Education Program has also developed a partnership of multiple stakeholder groups, which in addition to physicians includes patient-focused groups, such as the American Diabetes Association and others.

Voluntary Efforts at Standardization

Organizations that produce guidelines conduct their work and communicate their findings in different ways. Evidence-based guideline producers typically provide summary information about key findings including the quality of the individual studies included in the assessment, the quality of the overall body of evidence, and the strength of the recommendations. Each of these components can be depicted in a variety of ways by using letters, numbers, symbols, and words (Schünemann et al., 2003). For example, Table 5-2 highlights the grading scales that different organizations use to characterize the same cardiology interventions.

Although the overall quality of clinical practice guidelines has been improved by the efforts that have been made to grade the quality of evidence and the strength of recommendations, according to some the proliferation in the number of grading systems has undermined the value of the grading exercise (Guyatt et al., 2006a). As a result, many people have called for the development of a system that would standardize these grading systems and rating scales. The use of a common approach to grading the strength of recommendations is considered a mechanism that could facilitate the critical appraisal of a guideline development panel's judgments and aid the interpretation of the benefits and risks of an intervention (Guyatt et al., 2006a; Schünemann et al., 2006). Standardization is likely to be difficult, though, because many organizations have invested considerable time and effort in developing unique rating systems and are reluctant to change (Guyatt et al., 2006b).

A number of national and international programs use or are developing standardized grading scales within their organizations, including the USPSTF, the United Kingdom's NICE, and others (Schünemann et al., 2006). In addition, the major family medicine journals in the United States have created the Strength of Recommendation Taxonomy, which they be-

TABLE 5-2 Dueling Evidence Hierarchies and Recommendation Grades in Cardiology

Intervention and Organization	Quality of the Evidence	Strength of the Recommendation
Therapy for oral anticoagulation in patients with atrial fibrillation and rheumatic mitral valve disease		
American Heart Association	Level B	Class I
Scottish Intercollegiate Guidelines Network	Level 4	Grade C
American College of Chest Physicians	Grade C+	Grade 1C+
Implantable Cardioverter-Defibrillator therapy for cardiac arrest due to sustained ventricular fibrillation or ventricular tachycardia		
American College of Cardiology/American Heart Association	Level A	Class I
Scottish Intercollegiate Guidelines Network	Level 3/4	Grade D
European Society of Cardiology	Level B	Class IIa
Carotid endarterectomy for internal carotid artery stenosis or symptomatic stenosis		
American College of Cardiology/American Heart Association	Level C	Class IIa
American Academy of Neurology	Class I/II	Level A/B
Veterans Health Administration	Level I	Grade A

SOURCE: NGC (2007d); Schünemann et al. (2003).

lieve serves the needs of their specialty. Under that system, evidence from individual studies is rated as Level 1, 2, or 3; bodies of evidence are referred to as consistent or inconsistent; and the strength of recommendations are indicated by the letter A, B, or C (Ebell et al., 2004).

In addition to making efforts to reach agreement on grading scales, several groups have sought to standardize guideline development methodologies. Although there is still no internationally accepted standard for guideline development, there have been repeated calls for a "guideline for guidelines" (Guyatt et al., 2006b; Jackson and Feder, 1998; Schünemann et al., 2006; Shaneyfelt et al., 1999; Shekelle et al., 1999; Shiffman et al., 2003).

Among the more prominent efforts to standardize and raise the quality of clinical practice guidelines are the Appraisal of Guidelines Research and Evaluation (AGREE) collaboration and the Conference on Guideline Standardization (COGS). The AGREE collaboration defines the quality of guidelines as "the confidence that the potential biases inherent of guideline development have been addressed adequately and that the recommendations are both internally and externally valid, and are feasible for practice"

(The AGREE Collaboration, 2001). The AGREE instrument for assessing the quality of clinical practice guidelines is a result of an international collaboration that originated in Europe in 1998.

COGS convened in 2002 to define a set of standards for guidelines. Whereas the AGREE standards were developed as a means by which guidelines could be externally assessed after completion, the result of COGS was a tool for guideline developers to use as part of their work to improve the quality of their product. The COGS instrument provides a checklist of components necessary for the evaluation of guideline validity and usability (Shiffman et al., 2003). Both the AGREE instrument and the COGS checklist are included in Appendix F.

Adherence to Guidelines

Overall, the levels of adherence to guidelines and clinical recommendations vary greatly. While some guidelines are widely recognized and used (e.g., recommendations for infant sleeping position), others remain largely unnoticed. In rare instances, guidelines have become the center of media attention and controversy, such as mammography screening for breast cancer in women ages 40-49, in which guidelines differ as to whom should receive routine testing.

The rate of uptake of guidelines is increasing, but remains quite low. O'Malley and colleagues (2007) found that, over the period 1997 to 2005, the proportion of primary care physicians reporting that guidelines played a significant role in their decision making increased from 16 to 39 percent. Among specialists, these figures increased from 19 to 28 percent. The increases reported in the study were attributed to increasing access to health information technology and a greater link between adherence to guidelines and payment.

Lack of adherence to guidelines is reflective of the considerable practice variation that exists nationwide and is indicative of the fact that too often medical practice does not reflect much of what is known about effective clinical care (Reinertsen, 2003; Wennberg, 2004). However, the move toward performance measurement, pay-for-performance strategies, provider efficiency profiling, and electronic decision support is changing this dynamic promoting greater accountability for treatment decisions.

Limiting Factors

The decision to follow practice guidelines is voluntary, limiting the likelihood of universal adoption; as some have noted, guidelines are only guidelines (Cook and Giacomini, 1999). Limited adherence to guidelines reflects a number of factors, including a lack of physician awareness, a lack of agreement, and inertia (Cabana et al., 1999). Moreover, there are general concerns regarding the applicability of guidelines at the individual level. Guidelines are meant to define practices that meet the needs of most patients under most circumstances (Hunt et al., 2001). They aggregate the harms and benefits of interventions across a group of patients defined by clinical criteria rather than to individual patients.

In addition, they often focus on interventions related to a single condition and individual studies covered by the systematic reviews underpinning the guideline may exclude patients with multiple comorbidities (O'Connor, 2005). Practice guidelines may also apply to only a limited subset of the population and not address the needs of groups such as the elderly (Boyd et al., 2005). And, as described earlier, interpreting multiple guidelines on the same clinical topic may be difficult especially when there is contradictory guidance.

Local Translation

Tierney (2001) argues that guidelines, no matter how well crafted, must undergo "local translation" to be relevant and consistent with local clinical practice standards. However, this type of translation process may lock in some of the local variation that the guidelines are meant to reduce. Generally, to gain wide acceptance, physicians must accept guidelines as best practice (Ayanian et al., 1998; Fried et al., 2006). Yet physicians often do not agree that the standards being promoted through clinical practice guidelines represent the best course of action for their patients (Cabana et al., 1999). In fact, some physicians have accused guidelines of being invalid, unreliable, and irrelevant (Grilli et al., 2000).

Guideline Updates

Guidelines have limited shelf-lives given the rapid accumulation of new scientific knowledge and changes in practice stemming from new medical technologies and other advances. A review that looked at 17 guidelines published by the AHCPR in the 1990s estimated that about half of the guidelines had become outdated after 5.8 years (Shekelle et al., 2001). The authors concluded that guidelines be reassessed for their validity every 3 years.

To stay current, the organizations that issue guidelines must monitor the medical literature and be prepared to update the guideline. This standard is currently enforced by the NGC, which will not retain the guidelines in its database unless they have been developed, reviewed, or revised within the last 5 years.

CRITICAL PROGRAM CHALLENGES AND RECOMMENDATIONS

Building on the Current System

Efforts to improve the quality and availability of clinical practice guidelines need not involve a wholesale restructuring of the current system. The recommendations proposed by the committee build on the aspects of the current system that are functioning well—including the work of the USPSTF, the ACC/AHA, and others—but seek to raise the standards for producers of clinical practice guidelines overall.

Building on the current system is practical for a number of reasons. First, the experience of the AHCPR in the 1990s exposed the significant political risks involved in establishing government-sponsored clinical practice guidelines. When an AHCPR Patient Outcomes Research Team developed a guideline on the treatment of back pain, an angry group of orthopedic surgeons almost succeeded in convincing Congress to defund the agency (Gray, 1992; Gray et al., 2003). In addition, the private organizations that currently produce guidelines, such as professional societies and others, treasure their autonomy and would likely oppose efforts to reduce their role. Furthermore, guidelines that have the imprimatur of a respected professional society engender trust by the end users (Tunis et al., 1994). Finally, there are some indications that the quality of these guidelines has improved over time (Jackson and Feder, 1998), although data need to be updated. For these reasons, the committee believes that the pragmatic approach—and also the most promising approach—is to build on the current system.

Common Standards

Clinical practice guidelines vary widely in their methodological rigor and protection from bias; however, in the current environment, the organizations and individuals who use guidelines have very limited means to assess their objectivity or accuracy. The committee recommends several steps to ensure that the information communicated through practice guidelines is trustworthy.

Recommendation: Groups developing clinical guidelines or recommendations should use the Program's standards, document their adherence to the standards, and make this documentation publicly available.

The committee recommends that guideline development organizations adhere to a common set of standards that address the structure, process, reporting, and final product that contains the guidelines. Ensuring adherence to these standards, in part through public disclosure of adherence data, will increase the quality and accuracy of guidelines, as well as end users' confidence in adopting them. Thus, common standards will contribute to the overall success of the Program.

Although a number of consensus approaches to guideline standardization currently exist, there is not agreement on a single set of standards. The Program should develop (or endorse) standards for creating clinical practice guidelines, either by convening a panel of experts or by commissioning an outside group to perform this work. Below are a number of key standards that the committee believes will be important.

Standards of Critical Importance

Objectivity   Central to the development of effective guidelines is ensuring that the process is performed in an objective and impartial manner and that the conclusions are objective and impartial. Instituting balanced panel participation and governance will help to ensure that the clinical guidance that is produced is trustworthy. A more detailed discussion of the management of bias in guideline production follows later in this chapter.

Transparency   An important mechanism to promote trust is having a process that is open to the public. Conflicts of interest that may exist at the level of the panelist, panel, or sponsoring organization should be publicly disclosed. Deliberations that are open to the public and encourage public participation will ensure that a wide variety of perspectives are considered. Posting draft guidelines for public comment can also help achieve a greater balance of viewpoints.

The methods that the panel employs to gather, assess, and weigh evidence, as well as the mechanism that it uses to grade the strength of recommendations, should be explicitly defined, consistently applied, and available for public review. Of particular salience is the need to standardize, to the extent possible, the methods that the panels apply in the face of insufficient evidence.

Efficiency and timeliness   As the work of guideline producers becomes strategically aligned with national needs for improved information at the point of care, it is crucial that the work of these organizations be carried out in a timely fashion. Currently, patients and providers often make decisions in the absence of guidance in cases in which evidence reviews and practice guidelines have not been completed. Likewise, health plans and purchasers must make rapid coverage decisions regardless of whether or not guidelines are available.

To increase the volume of work that the system can produce overall, guideline developers should take steps to avoid the unnecessary duplication of effort and should deploy limited resources effectively. The Program should play a role in improving coordination among these activities. Improvements in cross-organizational efficiency can help ensure that technologies, procedures, and interventions are evaluated in a more timely fashion.

External review   Peer review conducted by outside experts is an important measure that can help ensure the quality of the guidelines produced. Groups that develop guidelines should institute a peer review process, in addition to allowing stakeholders and the public to review draft guidance. Organizations should adopt processes that include independent oversight of their responses to the peer review comments to ensure that they are responding appropriately to well-supported criticism.

Currency   Guidelines have limited shelf-lives as a result of the expanding evidence base and the corresponding changes in how medicine is practiced. Monitoring the medical literature for new evidence is an obligation of guideline developers. Organizations should not develop guidelines unless they are willing to keep them up to date.

Overlaps and gaps   To meet the needs of key decision makers, guideline producers must be aware that the conclusions offered by various recommending groups may often conflict. Voluntary efforts to promote consensus in specific topic areas should be a high priority. An important role for the Program will be identifying conflicts and convening efforts to resolve them. Groups that develop guidelines should be willing to participate in the reconciliation of their work with that of other groups when the need arises. In addition, processes for identifying and addressing the absence of guidelines for rare diseases and other clinical areas should also be established.

Common Language

The committee believes that a common language that expresses the strength of clinical practice recommendations should be an essential feature of the guideline development and reporting process. The use of a common language for all clinical practice recommendations is an efficient way to communicate the strength of evidence and assist end users with assessing the outputs of the various organizations that produce guidelines. This common language should convey the same information about the strength of evidence irrespective of the clinical service under consideration. In other words, guideline developers must use the same terms to describe the same quality of evidence for all clinical services.

Judgment about the strength of a recommendation derives from consideration of the benefits anticipated if the recommendation is followed and consideration of the potential harms and costs of such adherence. Strong recommendations are made when the benefits clearly exceed the harms or when the harms clearly exceed the benefits. On the contrary, lower-level recommendations (sometimes referred to as clinical "options") are made when the balance of the anticipated benefits compared with the anticipated harms and costs is less clear-cut or is essentially equivalent.

As mentioned above, the statement of the strength of the recommendation communicates an expectation regarding adherence. Whereas clinicians should be expected to follow strong recommendations unless a clear and compelling rationale for not doing so is present, patient preferences should also have a substantial role in influencing clinical decision making, and may even sometimes choose not to proceed with an intervention that has been found to be strongly beneficial. In addition, pay-for-performance measures should be built from strong recommendations and not clinical options.

The quality of the evidence (based on factors related to minimizing bias such as study design, consistency, and directness of the evidence) helps determine the confidence that should be placed in the balance equation. The guideline developer can confidently and strongly recommend an intervention when it is found effective and with minimal adverse effects in multiple, well-designed studies. Under such circumstances, one can be confident of the importance of adherence to the guideline. On the other hand, when high-quality evidence indicates both important benefits and important harms, the recommendation should be made accordingly. Strong recommendations should not be created when the evidence is poor. Nor should high-quality evidence on effectiveness automatically lead to a strong recommendation; potential harm must also be considered.

The committee believes that a common language that describes both the quality of the underlying evidence and the strength of recommendations is an important tool for promoting greater consistency among clinical practice guideline developers. This common language will reduce the requirements placed on end users in sorting through and navigating all the various terms, symbols, and expressions that currently exist. An important task for the Program will be to facilitate the process of achieving a common language.

Minimizing Bias Due to Conflicts of Interest

Organizations that produce guidelines convene panels of experts to assess the available evidence and develop clinical recommendations. To produce objective, well-balanced, reliable clinical guidance, guideline developers must address several basic structural issues that, if they are not managed properly, can create the perception—if not the reality—of bias.

These can diminish the value of the clinical information provided and can undermine public confidence in the guidelines overall.

Unbiased Information

Bias can enter into the guideline development process in a number of ways, as illustrated in Box 5-2. These biases can occur at the individual, panel, and organizational levels. Groups and organizations that develop clinical practice guidelines should address each of these to ensure that the end users view their guidelines as credible and trustworthy.

The committee identified and compared three approaches for handling conflicts of interest. The first is a permissive approach by which guideline producers are able to address these issues as they fit on a case-by-case basis. The current system is relatively permissive in how it handles potential conflicts, although some measures are in place to limit influence, such as restrictions on money or other gifts received from commercial sources that are placed on external advisors by the FDA and the NIH. Investigative reporting conducted by the print media has called into question guideline producers that have received industry financing, and this has raised public awareness. In addition, financial disclosures have increasingly been employed to address conflict of interest, and while this is an important step, its effectiveness may be limited. Moreover, guideline developers do not always disclose potential conflicts and biases that may exist at the individual, panel, or organizational level.

BOX 5-2
Potential Sources of Bias in Clinical Practice Guidelines

- Panelists have material interests in the recommendations, e.g., stock ownership, royalties, or other returns.
- Panelists have indirect financial interests, e.g., they could be paid for the health service under review or receive honoraria for discussing it.
- The panel is primarily made up of individuals from one specialty with only limited participation by other types of providers, patients, plans, methodologists, etc.
- Panelists have intellectual biases, e.g., prior research, strongly held opinions, or professional specialty that might compromise one's objectivity or bring it into question.
- The organization producing the guideline receives funding from companies with a material interest in the recommendations.
- The panel does not allow participation from members of the public.
- Panels do not allow participation from members of the public.

The second approach is to promote a system that is completely free from conflict of interest. Under such a system, panelists who had received any remuneration from affected industries would be disqualified from serving on guideline development panels. The restriction would also be applied to physicians who receive fee-for-service compensation for doing the procedures being reviewed. Presumably salaried physicians or physicians who do not provide the procedure themselves would qualify as panelists. Intellectual conflicts of interest, such as those relating to professional reputation, would also have to be addressed. At the organizational level, groups sponsored or convened by potentially affected manufacturers (including professional societies, consumer advocacy groups, and others) would not be recognized as appropriate sponsors of clinical practice guidelines.

Given the extent to which these types of conflicts exist in the current environment, the second "pure" model seems largely impractical. Guideline producers require panelists who have expertise and, in today's environment, these experts typically have conflicts of interest. Therefore, the committee identified a third, more pragmatic approach that recognizes that conflicts of interest are likely to persist for members of most guideline production panels, but that a number of steps can be taken to manage these conflicts. These steps include placing limits on the financial remuneration that panelists and organizations receive, balancing the composition of panels, and establishing a transparent process that includes public participation.

Table 5-3 illustrates measures that might be taken under each of the

TABLE 5-3 Measures to Address Conflicts of Interest

Approach	Panelist	Panel	Organization
Permissive	• Discretion of guideline producer	• Discretion of guideline producer	• Discretion of guideline producer
Pure	• No remuneration from affected manufacturers • Individuals with conflicts restricted to brief panel presentations	• Balanced panel participation (various provider/ stakeholder types, including plans, patients, and others)	• Guideline-producing organization receives no payments from affected manufacturers
Pragmatic	• Limited remuneration from affected manufacturers • Disclosure of conflicts • Publication of disclosed conflicts (transparency) • Limited voting rights for members with conflicts • Open (public) meetings	• Balanced panel participation (various provider/ stakeholder types, including plans, patients, and others)	• Guideline-producing organization receives limited payments from affected manufacturers

three approaches (permissive, pure, and pragmatic), across the various levels of the guideline production process (individual panelist, entire panel, and sponsoring organization). The permissive and the pure categories are intended to represent the extreme ends of the spectrum.

The committee maintains that the pragmatic approach is the most appropriate course of action, given that the current, more permissive approach provides too few safeguards against conflicts of interest and bias and that the "pure" approach, although it is theoretically desirable, is impractical and would strip too much expertise from the guideline development process. However, the Program, as detailed in Chapter 6, should develop (or endorse) strict standards to protect against bias and ensure that clinical practice guideline producers are adhering to these standards. In particular, the committee identified the following measures as a means of improving the quality of the information provided by guideline developers:

Recommendation: To minimize bias due to conflicts of interest, panels should include a balance of competing interests and diverse stakeholders, publish conflict of interest disclosures, and prohibit voting by members with material conflicts.

Individual Level

At the individual level, guideline developers should vet potential panelists for financial or intellectual biases and should have panelists disclose all financial relationships with commercial companies. They should also reveal any relevant positions that the panelists have advocated publicly. The Program should establish parameters to indicate when personal conflicts of interest are significant enough to warrant disqualification from panel participation or voting.

Panel Level

At the panel level, groups should be multidisciplinary and should include topic experts, generalists, consumers, payers (e.g., health plans), and others. For example, recommendations on care for children with Attention Deficit Hyperactivity Disorder should be developed with representation from pediatrics, family practice nursing, psychiatry and behavioral medicine, educators, parent organizations, and payers. Organizations should seek to build a broad consensus about the treatment alternatives that fall within the scope of the review. Purchasers and health plan representatives should be included on guideline development panels to moderate any clinical or manufacturer bias in favor of greater service utilization. In general, the panel should represent a balance of competing interests to the greatest extent possible.

Organizational Level

At the organizational level, guideline developers should disclose the monies they have received from affected manufacturers, either related to the subject of guideline development or any general contributions. The standards generated by the Program should establish the levels of commercial involvement or support at which organizations should be considered insufficiently protected from commercial bias.

Adherence to Standards

The end users of clinical guidelines and recommendations—physicians, performance measurement groups, health plans, purchasers, patients, policy makers, and others—would benefit from a rigorous set of development standards and a common reporting language that would improve the quality and usability of the guidelines. However, achieving this objective will be difficult. Various groups have developed distinct ways to speak about and assess evidence, and to grade the strength of their recommendations. Moreover, the rigors of their processes are highly variable; and many guideline developers do not have the resources or the ability to meet a set of structure, process, and product standards that are externally imposed.

Nevertheless, ensuring the quality and the usability of the information provided in clinical practice guidelines is vital to the performance of the health system and there is a need to promote compliance with these new guideline standards. Given the impracticality of centralizing the guideline development process in the U.S. government, the committee believes that building on the current pluralistic system is the most appropriate course of action. The committee proposes that the users of guidelines serve as the primary arbiters of guideline quality, with guideline developers voluntarily providing documentation that will allow end users to make informed judgments.

> **Recommendation: Providers, public and private payers, purchasers, accrediting organizations, performance measurement groups, patients, consumers, and others should preferentially use clinical recommendations developed according to the Program standards.**

The committee envisions that the Program will develop a common reporting mechanism that will enable guideline developers to describe the features of their process. Through a standardized survey instrument, guideline developers will be asked to report on their methodologies and their adherence to the common standards.

Guideline-producing organizations, spurred by end users, will want to include this documentation as part of the guideline itself. In addition, the information will be uploaded to a public web page to enable end users to view the extent to which organizations producing guidelines (and the guidelines themselves) adhere to the common standards. If guideline users preferentially adopt guidelines that are developed according to Program standards, guideline producers will be motivated to adhere to those standards and to provide documentation about their processes.

The availability of this information will enable the end users of the guideline material to become more informed about the quality of the information they receive. Although the documentation that guideline developers provide may not be complete, gaps in that information may serve as a red flag for the end users. In addition, through increased transparency and openness in the guideline development process, the accuracy of the information reported will be more easily verified.

The Program may want to consider instituting a certification or accreditation process to assure that specific guidelines or organizations developing them adhere to specific standards. Such an accreditation or certification process would allow for continued decentralized guideline production.

The end users of guideline information then become the group that holds the guideline developers accountable for their work products. The vision of the committee is that performance measurement groups will primarily rely on the highest-quality information—as indicated by the standards reporting document—and establish measures that will encourage physicians to comply with these high-quality recommendations. Health plans and purchasers should also be selective in choosing only guidelines that adhere to standards and base performance-based programs only on these types of guidelines. Accreditation groups (e.g., the National Committee for Quality Assurance, the Utilization Review Accreditation Commission, and the Joint Commission) should assess the extent to which the groups that they monitor are relying on the highest-quality clinical practice guideline information. Through this mechanism, the committee believes that improvements in guideline quality and clinical effectiveness information can be achieved.

REFERENCES

The AGREE Collaboration. 2001. *The Appraisal of Guidelines for Research and Evaluation (AGREE) instrument*. London, UK: The AGREE Research Trust http://www.agreetrust.org/docs/AGREE_Instrument_English.pdf (accessed September 2007).

AHRQ (Agency for Healthcare Research and Quality). 2007. *U.S. Preventive Services Task Force ratings* http://www.ahrq.gov/clinic/uspstf07/ratingsv2.htm (accessed September 14, 2007).

American Academy of Pediatrics. 2007. *History of the Red Book®* http://aapredbook. aappublications.org/about/#hist (accessed October 23, 2007).

Atkins, D., P. A. Briss, M. Eccles, S. Flottorp, G. Guyatt, R. T. Harbour, S. Hill, R. Jaeschke, A. Liberati, N. Magrini, J. Mason, D. O'Connell, A. D. Oxman, B. Phillips, H. Schünemann, T. T. Edejer, G. E. Vist, R. D. Williams, and the GRADE Working Group. 2005a. Systems for grading the quality of evidence and the strength of recommendations II: Pilot study of a new system. *BMC Health Services Research* 5(1).

Atkins, D., J. Siegel, and J. Slutsky. 2005b. Making policy when the evidence is in dispute. *Health Affairs* 24(1):102-113.

Ayanian, J. Z., M. B. Landrum, S.-L. T. Normand, E. Guadagnoli, and B. J. McNeil. 1998. Rating the appropriateness of coronary angiography—Do practicing physicians agree with an expert panel and with each other? *New England Journal of Medicine* 338(26): 1896-1904.

Beghi, E. 2004. Efficacy and tolerability of the new antiepileptic drugs: Comparison of two recent guidelines. *Lancet Neurology* 3(10):618-621.

Boyd, C. M., J. Darer, C. Boult, L. P. Fried, L. Boult, and A. W. Wu. 2005. Clinical practice guidelines and quality of care for older patients with multiple comorbid diseases: Implications for pay for performance. *JAMA* 294(6):716-724.

Boyd, E. A., and L. A. Bero. 2006. Improving the use of research evidence in guideline development: 4. Managing conflicts of interests. *Health Research Policy and Systems* 4(16).

Browman, G. P. 2001. Development and aftercare of clinical guidelines: The balance between rigor and pragmatism. *JAMA* 286(12):1509-1511.

Burgers, J. 2003. Characteristics of high-quality guidelines. *International Journal of Technology Assessment in Health Care* 19(1):148-157.

Burgers, J. S., and J. J. van Everdingen. 2004. Beyond the evidence in clinical guidelines. *The Lancet* 364(9432):392-393.

Cabana, M. D., C. S. Rand, N. R. Powe, A. W. Wu, M. H. Wilson, P.-A. C. Abboud, and H. R. Rubin. 1999. Why don't physicians follow clinical practice guidelines?: A framework for improvement. *JAMA* 282(15):1458-1465.

Campbell, E. G., R. L. Gruen, J. Mountford, L. G. Miller, P. D. Cleary, and D. Blumenthal. 2007. A national survey of physician-industry relationships. *New England Journal of Medicine* 356(17):1742-1750.

Choudhry, N. K., H. T. Stelfox, and A. S. Detsky. 2002. Relationships between authors of clinical practice guidelines and the pharmaceutical industry. *JAMA* 287(5):612-617.

Cook, D., and M. Giacomini. 1999. The trials and tribulations of clinical practice guidelines. *JAMA* 281(20):1950-1951.

Druss, B. G., and S. C. Marcus. 2005. Growth and decentralization of the medical literature: Implications for evidence-based medicine. *Journal of the Medical Library Association* 93(4):499-501.

Ebell, M., J. Siwek, B. D. Weiss, S. H. Woolf, J. Susman, B. Ewingman, and M. Bowman. 2004. Strength of Recommendation Taxonomy (SORT): A patient-centered approach to grading evidence in medical literature. *American Family Physician* 69(3):548-556.

Eddy, D. M. 2005. Evidence-based medicine: A unified approach. *Health Affairs* 24(1):9-17.

Fielding, J. E., and P. A. Briss. 2006. Promoting evidence-based public health policy: Can we have better evidence and more action? *Health Affairs* 25(4):969-978.

Fried, M., M. Farthing, J. Krabshuis, and E. Quigley. 2006. Global guidelines: Is gastroenterology leading the way? *Lancet* 368(9552):2041-2042.

GRADE Working Group. 2004. Grading quality of evidence and strength of recommendations. *BMJ* 328(7454):1490.

Gray, B. H. 1992. The legislative battle over health services research. *Health Affairs* 11(4): 38-66.

Gray, B. H., M. K. Gusmano, and S. Collins. 2003. AHCPR and the changing politics of health services research. *Health Affairs* w3.283.

Grilli, R., N. Magrini, A. Penna, G. Mura, and A. Liberati. 2000. Practice guidelines developed by specialty societies: The need for critical appraisal. *Lancet* 355:103-106.

Grimshaw, J. M., and I. T. Russell. 1993. Effect of clinical guidelines on medical practice: A systematic review of rigorous evaluations. *Lancet* 342:1317-1322.

Guirguis-Blake, J., N. Calonge, T. Miller, A. Siu, S. Teutsch, and E. Whitlock for the U.S. Preventive Services Task Force 2007. Current processes of the U.S. Preventive Services Task Force: Refining evidence-based recommendation development. *Annals of Internal Medicine* 0000605-200707170-200700170.

Guyatt, G., D. Gutterman, M. H. Baumann, D. Addrizzo-Harris, E. M. Hylek, B. Phillips, G. Raskob, S. Z. Lewis, and H. Schünemann. 2006a. Grading strength recommendations and quality of evidence in clinical guidelines: Report from an American College of Chest Physicians task force. *Chest* 129(1):174-181.

Guyatt, G., G. Vist, Y. Falck-Ytter, R. Kunz, N. Magrini, H. Schünemann, and R. Elena. 2006b. An emerging consensus on grading recommendations? *ACP Journal Club* A8-A9.

Harris, G., B. Carey, and J. Roberts. 2007. Psychiatrists, children and drug industry's role. *The New York Times*, "Health" http://www.nytimes.com/2007/05/10/health/10psyche. html?ei=5070&en= a90e19408d5df0cd&ex=1188964800&adxnnl=1&adxnnlx=11888 45745-KhpszR5rlQnw7Dxp8FR0Pw (accessed May 10, 2007).

Hasenfeld, R., and P. G. Shekelle. 2003. Is the methodological quality of guidelines declining in the U.S.? Comparison of the quality of U.S. Agency for Health Care Policy and Research (AHCPR) guidelines with those published subsequently. *Quality and Safety in Health Care* 12(6):428-434.

Hunt, S. A., D. W. Baker, M. H. Chin, M. P. Cinquegrani, A. M. Feldmanmd, G. S. Francis, T. G. Ganiats, S. Goldstein, G. Gregoratos, M. L. Jessup, R. J. Noble, M. Packer, M. A. Silver, L. W. Stevenson, R. J. Gibbons, E. M. Antman, J. S. Alpert, D. P. Faxon, V. Fuster, G. Gregoratos, A. K. Jacobs, L. F. Hiratzka, R. O. Russell, and S. C. Smith, Jr. 2001. ACC/AHA guidelines for the evaluation and management of chronic heart failure in the adult: Executive summary a report of the American College of Cardiology/ American Heart Association Task Force on Practice Guidelines (Committee to Revise the 1995 Guidelines for the Evaluation and Management of Heart Failure). *Circulation* 104(24):2996-3007.

IOM (Institute of Medicine). 1990. *Clinical practice guidelines: Directions for a new program.* Edited by Field, M. J., and K. N. Lohr. Washington, DC: National Academy Press.

———. 1992. *Guidelines for clinical practice: From development to use.* Edited by Field, M. J., and K. N. Lohr. Washington, DC: National Academy Press.

Jackson, R., and G. Feder. 1998. Guidelines for clinical guidelines. *BMJ* 317(7156):427-428.

Kahan, J. P., R. E. Park, L. L. Leape, S. J. Bernstein, L. H. Hilborne, L. Parker, C. J. Kamberg, D. J. Ballard, and R. H. Brook. 1996. Variations by specialty in physician ratings of the appropriateness and necessity of indications for procedures. *Medical Care* 34(6):512-523.

Kassirer, J. P. 2007. Chapter 7: Medicine's obsession with disclosure of financial conflicts: Fixing the wrong problem. In *Science and the media: Delgado's brave bulls and the ethics of scientific disclosure.* Edited by Snyder, P. J., L. Mayes, and D. Spencer. San Diego, CA: Academic Press, an imprint of Elsevier, Inc.

Miller, J., and J. Petrie. 2000. Development of practice guidelines. *Lancet* 355(9198):82-83.

Murphy, M. K., N. A. Black, D. L. Lamping, C. M. McKee, C. F. B. Sanderson, J. Askham, and T. Marteau. 1998. Consensus development methods, and their use in clinical guideline development. *Health Technology Assessment* 2(3):i-88.

NGC (National Guideline Clearinghouse). 2007a. *About inclusion criteria* http://www. guideline.gov/about/inclusion.aspx (accessed August 17, 2007).

————. 2007b. *Guideline index* http://www.guideline.gov/browse/guideline_index.aspx (accessed September 14, 2007).

————. 2007c. *NGC browse—organizations* http://www.guideline.gov/browse/browseorgsbyLtr. aspx?Letter=* (accessed June 2, 2007).

————. 2007d. *Search for cardiology* http://www.guideline.gov/search/searchresults.aspx? Type=3&txtSearch=cardiology&num=500 (accessed July 11, 2007).

————. 2007e. *Search for hypertension* http://www.guideline.gov/search/searchresults.aspx? Type=3&txtSearch=hypertension&num=500 (accessed August 12, 2007).

————. 2007f. *Search for stroke* http://www.guideline.gov/search/searchresults.aspx?Type=3 &txtSearch=stroke&num=500 (accessed August 12, 2007).

O'Connor, P. J. 2005. Adding value to evidence-based clinical guidelines. *JAMA* 294(6): 741-743.

O'Malley, A. S., H. H. Pham, and J. D. Reschovsky. 2007. Predictors of the growing influence of clinical practice guidelines. *Journal of General Internal Medicine* 22(6):742.

Perlin, J. B., and J. Kupersmith. 2007. Information technology and the inferential gap. *Health Affairs* 26(2):w192-w194.

Reinertsen, J. L. 2003. Zen and the art of physician autonomy maintenance. *Annals of Internal Medicine* 138(12):992-995.

Ricci, S., M. G. Celani, and E. Righetti. 2006. Development of clinical guidelines: Methodological and practical issues. *Neurological Sciences* 27(3):S228-S230.

Schünemann, H. J., D. Best, G. Vist, A. D. Oxman, and the GRADE Working Group. 2003. Letters, numbers, symbols and words: How to communicate grades of evidence and recommendations. *Canadian Medical Association Journal* 169(7):677-680.

Schünemann, H. J., A. Fretheim, and A. D. Oxman. 2006. Improving the use of research evidence in guideline development: 9. Grading evidence and recommendations. *Health Research Policy and Systems* 4(21).

Schwartz, J. S. 1984. The role of professional medical societies in reducing practice variations. *Health Affairs* 3(2):90-101.

Shaneyfelt, T. M., M. F. Mayo-Smith, and J. Rothwangl. 1999. Are guidelines following guidelines?: The methodological quality of clinical practice guidelines in the peer-reviewed medical literature. *JAMA* 281(20):1900-1905.

Shekelle, P. G., S. H. Woolf, M. Eccles, and J. Grimshaw. 1999. Clinical guidelines: Developing guidelines. *BMJ* 318(7183):593-596.

Shekelle, P. G., E. Ortiz, S. Rhodes, S. C. Morton, M. P. Eccles, J. M. Grimshaw, and S. H. Woolf. 2001. Validity of the Agency for Healthcare Research and Quality clinical practice guidelines: How quickly do guidelines become outdated? *JAMA* 286(12):1461-1467.

Shiffman, R. N., P. Shekelle, M. Overhage, J. Slutsky, J. Grimshaw, and A. M. Deshpande. 2003. Standardized reporting of clinical practice guidelines: A proposal from the Conference on Guideline Standardization. *Annals of Internal Medicine* 139(6):493-500.

Stelfox, H. T. 1998. Conflict of interest in the debate over calcium-channel antagonists. *New England Journal of Medicine* 338(2):101-106.

Stewart, W. F., N. R. Shah, M. J. Selna, R. A. Paulus, and J. M. Walker. 2007. Bridging the inferential gap: The electronic health record and clinical evidence. *Health Affairs* 26(2): w181-w191.

Thomson, R., H. McElroy, and M. Sudlow. 1998. Guidelines on anticoagulant treatment in atrial fibrillation in Great Britain: Variation in content and implications for treatment. *BMJ* 316(7130):509-513.

Tierney, W. M. 2001. Improving clinical decisions and outcomes with information: A review. *International Journal of Medical Informatics* 62:1-9.

Tonelli, M. R. 2007. Conflict of interest in clinical practice. *Chest* 132(2):664-670.

077

Tunis, S. R., R. S. A. Hayward, M. C. Wilson, H. R. Rubin, E. B. Bass, M. Johnston, and E. P. Steinberg. 1994. Internists' attitudes about clinical practice guidelines. *Annals of Internal Medicine* 120(11):956-963.

Weinstein, J. N., K. Clay, and T. S. Morgan. 2007. Informed patient choice: Patient-centered valuing of surgical risks and benefits. *Health Affairs* 26(3):726-730.

Wennberg, J. E. 2004. Perspective: Practice variations and health care reform: Connecting the dots. *Health Affairs* var.140.

Woolf, S. H., and D. Atkins. 2001. The evolving role of prevention in health care: Contributions of the U.S. Preventive Services Task Force. *American Journal of Preventive Medicine* 20(3, S1):13-20.

Woolf, S. H., R. Grol, A. Hutchinson, M. Eccles, and J. Grimshaw. 1999. Clinical guidelines: Potential benefits, limitations, and harms of clinical guidelines. *BMJ* 318(7182):527-530.

6

Building a Foundation for Knowing What Works in Health Care

Abstract: The committee recommends that Congress direct the secretary of the U.S. Department of Health and Human Services to establish a single national clinical effectiveness assessment program ("the Program") with the authority and resources to set priorities for and sponsor systematic reviews of clinical effectiveness, and to develop methodologic and reporting standards for conducting systematic reviews and developing clinical guidelines. The secretary should appoint a broadly representative Clinical Effectiveness Advisory Board to oversee the Program. This chapter considers three alternative approaches to building the Program infrastructure: the status quo, a central agency model, and a hybrid model. In the previous chapters, the committee found convincing evidence that systematic reviews and clinical guidelines are often of poor quality, lacking scientific rigor and objectivity. The committee observed that, under the status quo, systematic reviews and clinical guidelines are produced by numerous public and private organizations with little or no coordination, minimal quality controls, inconsistent terminology, inadequate transparency, and without concerted attention to the priorities of all types of consumers, patients, and other stakeholders. The committee finds that in a highly centralized program, such as in a central agency, the quality of both evidence assessment and guideline development may be tightly controlled. But, such an agency would be costly and take too much time to establish. Thus, the committee recommends that the secretary build on existing capacity to establish the Program infrastructure (the hybrid approach), with substantial stakeholder involvement and strict standards to protect against bias and conflict of interest.

The United States must substantially strengthen its capacity for scientific inquiry into evidence on what is known and not known about what works in health care. Under the status quo, there is not enough objective and credible information identifying which health services work best, for whom, and under what circumstances (Medicare Payment Advisory Commission, 2007). Interest in a national comparative clinical effectiveness program is growing. Recently, the Medicare Payment Advisory Commission concluded unanimously that because information on clinical effectiveness can benefit all users and is a public good, the federal government should act to produce unbiased information and make it publicly available (Medicare Payment Advisory Commission, 2007). Other stakeholders and analysts agree (America's Health Insurance Plans, 2007; BCBSA, 2007b; Congressional Budget Office, 2007; IOM, 2007; Kupersmith et al., 2005; Shortell et al., 2007; Wilensky, 2006).

The previous chapters examined three essential functions—priority setting, evidence assessment (systematic review), and developing clinical practice guidelines—of a national clinical effectiveness assessment program ("the Program"). This chapter explores how best to approach establishing an infrastructure for organizing the three functions. It first reviews the foundational principles that the committee adopted to guide its analysis and then assesses three alternatives (i.e., the status quo, a central agency model, and a hybrid model). The chapter concludes with the committee's recommendations regarding the program infrastructure.

GUIDING PRINCIPLES

During the course of this study, a number of important themes emerged that led the committee to establish a set of guiding principles for building the Program. These themes include convincing evidence (described in the previous chapters) that financial and other types of conflicts of interest may compromise the integrity of research findings and related clinical recommendations, indications that a meaningful proportion of evidence reviews frequently lack scientific rigor, and current efforts fall far short of addressing patients' and health professionals' need for current, trustworthy information on clinical effectiveness. The committee particularly wants to ensure that its recommended Program will be stable over the long term, that its output be judged as objective and meeting broadly accepted standards of scientific rigor, that it will be useful to stakeholders, that it is without conflict of interest or bias,[1] and that its operations be independent of external political pressures.

---

[1]The term "bias" has different meaning depending on the context in which it is used. Here it refers to "bias" due to conflicts of interest. In discussions regarding systematic review methods,

In developing and defining its guiding principles, the committee also drew from important foundational work performed by others—most notably, several earlier Institute of Medicine (IOM) committees, including the Committee on Quality of Health Care in America, the Committee on Setting Priorities for Guidelines Development, and the Committee on Priorities for Assessment and Reassessment of Health Care Technologies; the Agency for Healthcare Research and Quality (AHRQ); the Cochrane Collaboration; the AGREE (Appraisal of Guidelines Research and Evaluation) Collaboration; the GRADE Working Group; and the National Quality Forum (AGREE Collaboration, 2001; AHRQ, 2007; Cochrane Collaboration, 2007; GRADE Working Group, 2004; IOM, 1992, 1995, 2001; NQF, 2006).

Box 6-1 defines eight guiding principles for organizing the Program: accountability, consistency, efficiency, feasibility, objectivity, responsiveness, scientific rigor, and transparency. The committee believes that each principle is integral to ensuring a valued, effective enterprise that instills credibility and trust in its products. The following sections further describe each principle.

Accountability

For the Program, accountability refers to accepting the responsibility to meet and demonstrate compliance with a set of program performance standards. Under the status quo, a meaningful proportion of systematic reviews of clinical effectiveness are proprietary and their findings are available only to those who pay for them. The documentation on the methods used to conduct systematic reviews is uneven and often lacking, even when the review and analysis are presented in a journal or some other public medium (Moher et al., 2007). As a result, it may be impossible to determine if the review process was free from bias and met scientific and performance standards.

Consistency

Consistency refers to the use of standardized and predictable methods. It is an important element not only in a program's regulations and administrative procedures, but also in its analytic methods and products. Although a number of organizations and individuals currently generate high-quality evidence syntheses, potential users of the information are often frustrated by unexplained differences in the terminologies, methods, and conclusions.

"bias" refers to statistical bias, i.e., the tendency for a study to produce results that systematically depart from the truth.

BOX 6-1
Program Principles

Accountability	Parties are directly responsible for meeting standards.
Consistency	Processes are predictable and standardized so as to be readily usable by patients, health professionals, medical societies, payers, and purchasers.
Efficiency	Avoids waste and unnecessary duplication.
Feasibility	Capable of operating in the real world; recognizing political, economic, and social implications.
Objectivity	Evidence-based and without bias, e.g., balanced participation, governance, and standards minimize conflicts of interest and other biases.
Responsiveness	Addresses information needs of decision makers in a timely way. Able to react quickly. Patients and health professionals require real-time, up-to-date information for treatment decisions.
Scientific rigor	Methods minimize bias, provide reproducible results, and are completely reported.
Transparency	Methods are explicitly defined, consistently applied, and available for public review so that observers can readily link judgments, decisions, or actions to the data on which they are based.

When reviews present methods and findings in a uniform way, it is easier for the user to appraise the evidence as a whole and assess the underlying differences in the findings from studies assessing a similar question. Another advantage of consistency is that it makes it easier for manufacturers to make accurate predictions of budgets for the evaluation of new technologies and new applications of existing technologies for product evaluation.

Efficiency

Efficiency means the avoidance of waste and the effective use of resources. Setting national priorities for which services should be evaluated can help avoid unnecessary duplication and can also focus limited resources on the most important questions. It is not efficient for every payer, provider organization, or medical professional society to invest in assessment of the same topics. Guideline developers and payers faced with coverage decisions are overburdened with duplicating production of systematic reviews. Numerous private sector organizations, such as health plans and technology assessment firms, set their own priorities for assessing evidence but their research is often duplicative as many parties tend to focus on the same set of emerging technologies and new applications of existing technologies (BCBSA, 2007a; ECRI, 2006; Hayes, 2006). While some duplication may be desirable and private organizations should be free to set their own research priorities, users of evidence have little basis for deciding which available reviews to rely upon.

Feasibility

For a program to be feasible it must be able to function in the real world; its processes must be sound, its resources must be adequate over the long term, and its leaders must pay attention to stakeholders. A program must also be attuned to political realities. If the program lacks sufficient public support, it will be neither implemented nor sustained. If the program is not protected from political conflict and funding is withdrawn, the public investment will be wasted and any gains made will be lost. This lesson has been repeated numerous times during the decades of on-and-off federal involvement in research on clinical effectiveness (Congressional Budget Office, 2007). In particular, the committee notes the experience of AHRQ as an example of political pressures that have short-circuited the important beginnings of high-quality clinical effectiveness research in the United States. In the early 1990s, funding for AHRQ was almost eliminated due to stakeholders' anger over the findings presented in its guideline on interventions for back pain (Gray, 1992; Gray et al., 2003).

Objectivity

Objectivity requires the incorporation of certain features in a program, such as balanced participation, governance, and standards that minimize conflicts of interest and other biases. Objectivity is central to the development of public confidence in the integrity of an organization. Patients, health professionals, payers, and developers of practice guidelines depend on systematic reviews to know whether the available evidence is valid. They need to be able to trust the Program to reach conclusions that are driven solely by the evidence and never by special interests that may benefit materially. The public will not trust a program that does not have adequate protections against bias and conflict of interest.

As the previous chapters have described, there is a growing literature documenting that in comparison with non-industry-sponsored research, industry-sponsored research—including evidence reviews—is more likely to favor the sponsor's product (Lexchin et al., 2003). Financial interests are not the only source of bias. Program participants may have intellectual biases (e.g., regarding their own body of work), or program processes may favor one professional specialty over another (e.g., surgery versus medicine, ophthalmology versus optometry).

Although it may not always be possible to make a process entirely free from bias, there are always steps that can be taken to address areas of concern. For example, many studies of devices and drugs are funded by their manufacturers. Given legitimate concerns about reporting biases, detailed information about funding sources should always be made public. Moreover, systematic reviews should indicate the funding source not only for the individual studies, but also for the review itself. The Program may find advice from a forthcoming report from the IOM Committee on Conflict of Interest in Medical Research, Education, and Practice. The committee is developing guidance for managing conflicts of interest in the development of clinical practice guidelines and conduct of medical research. A final report is expected in 2009.

Responsiveness

The overall value of the Program will hinge, in part, on how responsive it is to the information needs of decision makers, i.e., patients, clinicians, health plans, purchasers, specialty societies, and other decision makers. No mechanism currently insures that evidence assessments address the concerns of all types of patients or all types of services across the continuum of care. In many cases, evidence on effectiveness does not extend to children, older individuals, minority populations, people with multiple conditions, or particular community settings; and new research may be warranted (National Research Council, 2004; Simpson, 2004).

Responsiveness also implies timeliness including an obligation to stay current on the topics of research. The frequency with which reviews need updating depends on the production of valid new evidence. The Cochrane Collaboration recommends that systematic reviews be updated every two years or should have a commentary to explain why this is done less frequently. This recommendation has been supported by a recent study conducted by Shojania and colleagues (2007). The investigators analyzed the need for updates of 100 clinically relevant systematic reviews of drugs, devices, and procedures that signaled the need for an update, such as new trial evidence reversing the findings of an earlier effectiveness review. They found that almost one in four reviews (23 percent) needed an update within two years of publication of the reviews, 15 percent within one year, and 7 percent before publication.

Scientific Rigor

As applied to evidence reports and recommendation statements, scientific rigor implies that research methods minimize bias, that the results are reliable and valid, and that both the methods used and all results are completely reported. Methods have been developed for systematically reviewing evidence on effectiveness and these methods are evidence based (i.e., the evidence has shown that failure to adhere to these methods can result in invalid or biased findings) (Higgins and Green, 2006; Moher et al., 1999; Stroup et al., 2000). However, as noted earlier, there is considerable evidence indicating that many systematic reviews do not meet scientific standards (Gøtzsche et al., 2007; Moher et al., 2007). Particularly worrisome is the lack of attention to the quality and scientific rigor of the studies that are included in the review. Publication in a high-impact journal, unfortunately, does not guarantee that the methods used in the study were sound (Steinberg and Luce, 2005). Less is known about bias-free processes for translating evidence into clinical recommendations.

Transparency

In the present context, transparency refers to the use of clear, unambiguous language to convey scientific results and conclusions. It gives the reader the ability to clearly link judgments, decisions, or actions to the information on which they are based. Different entities frequently review the same published evidence and arrive at different conclusions about their safety and effectiveness, and it is important to be able to identify possible explanations. Methods should be explicitly defined, consistently applied, and available for public review so that observers can readily link judgments, decisions, or actions to the data on which they are based. There is extensive evidence that most systematic reviews lack adherence to a transparent and documented set of standards (Bhandari et al., 2001; Delaney et al., 2005; Glenny et al., 2003; Hayden et al., 2006; Jadad and McQuay, 1996; Jadad et al., 2000; Mallen et al., 2006; Moher et al., 2007; Whiting et al., 2005). This undermines the public's ability to be confident in the integrity of the process.

Reporting standards provide transparency by requiring extensive discussion on the methods used to conduct the review in sufficient detail to replicate the results. In 1999 and 2000, QUOROM (Quality of Reporting of Meta-analyses) and MOOSE (Meta-analysis Of Observational Studies in Epidemiology) reporting standards were published to improve the quality of meta-analyses, although neither set of standards has become widely adopted (Moher et al., 2007). CONSORT (Consolidated Standards for Reporting Trials) has simplified the task of summarizing evidence from randomized controlled trials (Moher et al., 1999; Stroup et al., 2000).

BUILDING THE PROGRAM'S FOUNDATION

This section considers how best to approach building the Program based on the foundational principles outlined above. The section begins with a brief review of programs in other countries and then examines three alternative models for the United States.

International Approaches to Identifying Effective Services

Many countries have developed programs to examine the effectiveness of clinical services. In Europe, 16 countries have at least one publicly affiliated agency responsible for assessing clinical effectiveness. Australia, Canada, and Singapore, among other countries, also have clinical effectiveness programs. As with the efforts made by various agencies and parties to assess clinical effectiveness in the United States, over the past three to four decades efforts elsewhere in the world have been prompted by concern with the high cost of medical interventions, as well as concern about the unsubstantiated benefits of widely disseminated clinical practices (Jonsson, 2002; Oliver et al., 2004).

The European Community (EC) has promoted priority setting, effectiveness assessments, and information sharing and the dissemination of results since 1994 (Velasco-Garrido and Busse, 2005). Health technology assessment has been a specific priority of the EC since 2004. The EC established the European Network for Health Technology Assessment (EUnetHTA) in 2006 to promote better coordination of national efforts (Kristensen and the EUnetHTA Partners, 2006). This Europe-wide initiative serves as an umbrella effort to make sure that there is no duplication of efforts and to bring up standards across individual countries and agencies.

Scope, Priority Setting, and Evidence Assessments
in Selected National Programs

Systematic, detailed information on the operations of most national clinical effectiveness programs is limited, and studies assessing and comparing the impacts of these programs are even more limited (Oliver et al., 2004). The documentation and evaluation of national programs assessing clinical effectiveness that are available point to both the growth in capacity over time and the need for processes that are more consistent, transparent, and evidence based (Draborg and Gyrd-Hansen, 2005; García-Altés et al., 2004; Velasco-Garrido and Busse, 2005). The committee has not undertaken an in-depth study of international models for developing knowledge about clinical effectiveness, and this brief overview does not endorse any country's particular approach.

TABLE 6-1 Focus of Selected National Efforts to Identify Effective Health Care Services

Country	Drugs	Devices[a]	Preventive Services	Surgical Procedures[b]
United States	✓	✓	✓	
Australia	✓	✓	✓	✓
Canada	✓	✓	✓	✓
Denmark	✓	✓	✓	✓
France	✓	✓	✓	✓
Germany	✓	✓	✓	✓
Scotland	✓	✓	✓	✓
England and Wales	✓	✓	✓	✓

[a]Includes diagnostic and therapeutic devices (e.g., ultrasound machines, stents, and inhaler devices).

[b]Includes the assessment of operating techniques, the use of surgical equipment for a specific procedure, and comparative effectiveness of surgical procedures.

SOURCE: Australian Safety & Efficacy Register of New Interventional Procedures-Surgical (2005); CADTH (2006); Canadian Task Force on Preventive Health Care (2005); Department on Health and Ageing (2006); Haute Autorité de Santé (2007); Institute for Quality and Efficiency in Health Care (2007); National Board of Health (2007); National Health and Medical Research Council (2006); NICE (2007); SIGN (2007).

The effectiveness review programs in Australia, Canada, Denmark, France, Germany, and the United Kingdom[2] assess a broad range of clinical services, including drugs, devices, tests, imaging procedures, preventive services, and surgical procedures (Table 6-1). The programs in Australia, Canada, Germany, and the United Kingdom assess both clinical effectiveness and cost-effectiveness (Table 6-2). In Australia, evidence of the comparative effectiveness of new drugs, devices, and procedures, including comparative cost-effectiveness, must be assessed before the national health insurance program will approve coverage. Manufacturers are required to submit extensive documentation on the effectiveness of their products to facilitate the assessment. In Canada, a national agency coordinates clinical and economic assessments and provides participating provincial and other public pharmaceutical benefits plans with coverage recommendations Canadian (CADTH, 2006). A governing board, composed of federal and regional health officials, selects which topics are to be assessed. In England and Wales, the National Institute for Health and Clinical Excellence (NICE), a special health authority within the National Health Service (NHS), assesses effectiveness. In Scotland, two organizations provide advice to the local health authorities within NHS Scotland: the Scottish Medicines

---

[2]England and Wales have a separate program from Scotland.

TABLE 6-2 Key Features of National Clinical Effectiveness Programs in Australia, Canada, and England and Wales

National Organization (Country)	Scope of Review	Entities That Select Topics and Set Priorities	Entities That Perform Evidence Assessments	Types of Decisions
Pharmaceutical Benefits Advisory Committee (Australia)	Comparative clinical and cost-effectiveness of drugs	Manufacturers seeking coverage of new drugs submit application for review.	Internal and external organizations. Manufacturers and other third parties must submit detailed applications to support coverage review.	Coverage (advisory to Minister of Health and Ageing)
Medical Services Advisory Committee (MSAC) (Australia)	Safety, effectiveness, and cost-effectiveness of new medical technologies and procedures	Medical profession, industry, or others seeking coverage for new medical technology or procedure submit application; MSAC prioritizes reviews.	External health technology assessment organizations advised by internal panels of MSAC members, experts, and consumers.	Coverage (advisory to Minister of Health and Ageing)
Canadian Agency for Drugs and Technologies in Health (Canada)	Clinical and cost-effectiveness of drugs, devices for diagnosis and treatment, procedures, and health services management	Board of Directors (Deputy Health Ministers from federal, provincial, and territorial health agencies) selects topics.	Internal and external organizations; activities of seven provincial health technology assessment organizations are coordinated.	Coverage recommendations for drugs; advisory for other services
NICE (England and Wales)	Clinical and cost-effectiveness of drugs, devices, diagnostics, surgical procedures, and health promotion interventions	Individuals and groups[a] may propose topics. Department of Health selects topics.	External groups perform initial assessment; expert committees are convened to do final assessment with internal staff support.[b]	Coverage, development of guidelines, and clinical audit methods

[a]Includes health professionals, patients and the general public, clinical directors within the Department of Health, manufacturers, and the National Horizon Scanning Centre of the University of Birmingham (a group that tracks emerging technologies).
[b]Manufacturers may submit an initial assessment, which is then reviewed and critiqued by an external review group.
SOURCE: Lopert (2006); Miller (2006); Sanders (2002).

Consortium, which reviews new drugs and new indications for the use of existing drugs for clinical effectiveness and cost-effectiveness, and the Scottish Intercollegiate Guidelines Network (SIGN), which develops and disseminates recommendations for effective clinical practices.

Relevance to the United States

The countries listed in Table 6-1 differ from the United States in that they have government-sponsored health coverage. Yet, none of those national programs supports a health system that exceeds the scope of current U.S. federal expenditures on health—an estimated $645 billion in 2005—for Medicare, Medicaid, the State Children's Health Insurance Program, the U.S. Department of Defense, the Veterans Health Administration, and the Indian Health Service. Moreover, the United States spends more per capita on health care than any other country. In 2002, U.S. per capita health spending was $5,267; 53 percent more than any other country (Anderson et al., 2005). Thus, despite smaller expenditure bases, these national systems have chosen to make substantial investments to identify the most effective clinical services and apply such knowledge to promote and improve health outcomes. Many of them also take explicit account of the cost-effectiveness of particular clinical services to conserve and optimize their programs' finite financial resources. Notably, these national systems use relatively centralized coverage-oriented programs both to improve the investment of public resources in health care (e.g., the Pharmaceutical Benefits Advisory Committee in Australia) and to ensure the availability of effective new technologies throughout a national system (e.g., NICE in England and Wales).

It is difficult to generalize about the impact of national technology assessment programs on the adoption of new clinical interventions. One recent study that examined the rates of diffusion of new clinical technologies in 10 countries found mixed results for the adoption of particular technologies across countries. Still, the presence of a clinical effectiveness report or some other form of guidance was consistently associated with the increased diffusion of the technology (as was above-average per capita spending on health care) (Packer et al., 2006).

Another insight from the international experience with programs that assess clinical effectiveness is that the mere development and publication of information, even by the most authoritative sources, are not in and of themselves sufficient to ensure changes in policy and practice (Battista, 2006; Oliver et al., 2004). National programs have moved in the direction of increasing the transparency of their assessment processes, placing a greater emphasis on the dissemination and communication of the results of assessments, and in some cases encouraging greater consumer involvement. In structuring a program uniquely suited to U.S. circumstances, the United

States can learn from the history of and progress that other countries have made.

Alternative Models for a U.S. National Clinical Effectiveness Assessment Program

The committee considered three approaches to establishing the Program infrastructure: maintaining the status quo and two alternatives (described below). Table 6-3 compares key aspects of the status quo with the two proposed alternatives: a central agency and a hybrid model. Both alterna-

TABLE 6-3 Alternative Approaches to Organizing the Program: Administrative Structure and Primary Functions

Organizational Feature or Function	Status Quo
Structure	
Administrative infrastructure	No change.
Degree of program control over clinical effectiveness assessment process	There is no change, except when sponsored by the AHRQ Effective Health Care Program.
Primary functions	
Setting research priorities	Multiple public and private entities set program- or mission-specific priorities. AHRQ sets priorities as directed by the secretary of the U.S. Department of Health and Human Services.
Assessing evidence	Multiple, independent organizations operating without oversight. No standardized mechanisms for quality assurance and quality control.
Developing clinical guidelines/recommendations	Multiple, independent organizations operating without oversight. Multiple, voluntary practice guidelines are available. No standardized mechanisms for quality assurance and quality control; claims of evidence base not necessarily supported by methods.

tives to the status quo would require that the Program substantially scale up resources, develop rigorous methodological and reporting standards (including common terminology), and institute protections against bias due to conflict of interest.

Status Quo

As the previous chapters described, the committee found convincing evidence that systematic reviews and clinical guidelines are often of poor quality, lacking scientific rigor and objectivity. Under the status quo, systematic reviews and clinical guidelines are produced by numerous public

Agency Model	Hybrid Approach
Infrastructure is sufficient to support significant expansion in evidence assessment and to develop standards for evidence assessments, clinical guidelines, and bias protections. Executive staff oversee the Program.	Infrastructure is sufficient to support significant expansion in and to develop standards for systematic reviews, clinical guidelines, and bias protections. An independent advisory board oversees the Program. Membership of the board includes diverse public and private sector expertise.
High. Mandatory standards and processes. In-house staff oversee and conduct key functions for priority setting, evidence reviews, and clinical recommendation development.	Mixed. Control over priority setting and to a large extent over systematic review functions, which must meet standards and bias protections. No direct control over clinical recommendation development, though standards set.
Agency establishes priorities for systematic reviews of clinical effectiveness and clinical guidelines. Process is based in statute and provides for public and stakeholder input.	Priority Setting Advisory Committee (PSAC) establishes priorities for systematic reviews of clinical effectiveness (with public and stakeholder input). The PSAC includes a broad mix of expertise and interests to minimize bias due to conflicts of interest.
Conducted by in-house staff and outside organizations in accordance with program standards. Stronger protections against bias.	Conducted in accordance with program standards. Stronger protections against bias.
Developed by in-house staff and outside organizations in accordance with program standards. Stronger protections against bias.	Multiple, independent organizations operating without oversight. Program promotes use of voluntary standards. No direct protections against bias in voluntary activities.

and private organizations with little or no coordination, minimal quality controls, inconsistent terminology, inadequate transparency, and without concerted attention to the priorities of all types of consumers, patients, and other stakeholders. Perhaps as a consequence, while many important topics remained unexamined, there is unnecessary duplication of effort in assessments of new and emerging technologies. No one agency or organization in the United States evaluates from a broad, national perspective the effectiveness of new as well as established health interventions for all populations, children as well as elderly people, women as well as men, and ethnic and racial minorities.

Central Agency Model

The first alternative to the status quo, coined the "central agency model," is a single, highly centralized entity, such as an executive branch agency or a division of an executive agency. It would have broad authority to fund, carry out, and control the full range of analytic tasks: setting priorities for systematic reviews, producing systematic reviews, and developing clinical guidelines—all in accordance with mandatory Program standards. Some or all of the Program's procedures could be based in statute (e.g., mandatory priority setting criteria). The agency would be led by executive-level staff who would oversee Program activities with support from an extensive Program staff.

Hybrid Model

The second alternative to the status quo, referred to as the "hybrid model," builds on current private and public sector capacity but gives the Program the authority and sufficient funding to develop process and reporting standards for, to set priorities for, and to sponsor standards-based systematic reviews of high-priority topics. The Program's role regarding clinical guideline development would be threefold: (1) developing (or endorsing) rigorous but voluntary guidelines standards, (2) promoting voluntary compliance with guideline standards, and (3) providing a forum for resolving conflicts between existing guidelines. An independent advisory board would oversee the Program. A group of core staff would be needed, but the Program would rely extensively on outside experts and organizations.

Comparing the Agency and Hybrid Models

Table 6-4 compares the committee's assumptions about the alternative models' likely adherence to the guiding principles outlined earlier in

TABLE 6-4 Summary Assessment of Organizational Alternatives Based on Committee Principles

Principles	Status Quo	Agency Model	Hybrid Model
	No change.	*Centralizes responsibility in an expanded or new agency, which determines priorities, and funds, produces, and sets mandatory standards and language for both systematic reviews and clinical recommendations/guidelines. Responsible for making clinical guidelines and recommendations.*	*A national Program determines priorities (with public input), funds, and sets mandatory standards and language for systematic reviews. External groups and individuals produce systematic reviews. Establishes voluntary standards for clinical recommendations/guidelines. Existing organizations produce clinical guidelines and recommendations.*
Accountability— *Parties are directly responsible for meeting and demonstrating compliance with minimum standards*	Poor. Systematic reviews and guidelines are often proprietary or available only to members. When publicly available, methods used often lack complete documentation.	Moderate to high. Central agency is directly responsible for and reports on compliance. Congress provides oversight.	*Moderate to high.* Program is directly responsible for priority setting and systematic reviews. Reliance on disclosure of compliance with common standards and end user preference for guidelines produced according to standards.
Consistency— *Standardized and predictable methods*	Poor. Systematic reviews and clinical recommendations may not use standardized, evidence-based methods.	*High.* Standardization of methods is accomplished with a unified management structure.	*Moderate to high.* Funding mechanism for systematic reviews requires standardization of methods. Reliance on disclosure of compliance with common standards and end user preference for guidelines produced according to standards.

continued

TABLE 6-4 Continued

Principles	Status Quo	Agency Model	Hybrid Model
Efficiency—*Avoids waste and unnecessary duplication*	*Poor.* Redundant and conflicting evidence reviews and guidelines are common.	*Moderate to high.* Depends on effective and well-targeted implementation.	*Moderate to high.* Unnecessary duplication of priority setting and systematic reviews is reduced. Potential for duplication of clinical recommendations remains.
Feasibility—*Capable of operating in the real world*	*High.* No change from current practice. But without additional funding, output will be relatively low or unpredictable from year to year.	*Poor.* Political support seems unlikely given high cost, new bureaucracy, and assumption of some responsibilities previously in the private sector (i.e., making clinical recommendations). Private sector organizations may strongly resist the agency's takeover of some of their current activities. Will require larger professional-technical workforce.	*Moderate.* Requires new or expanded infrastructure and increased expenditures. May face political resistance among some affected stakeholders. Will require larger professional-technical workforce but more will be accomplished.
Objectivity—*Evidence-based and without bias; conflict of interest is minimized*	*Poor.* Voluntary and conflicting standards, inconsistently applied.	*High.* Integrated process and autonomous operational structure supports enforcement of standards.	*Moderate to high.* Program products must meet common standards for conflict of interest, priority setting, and production of systematic reviews that minimize statistical bias. Reliance on disclosure of compliance with common standards and end user preference for guidelines produced according to standards.

Responsiveness— *Addresses information needs of decision makers (i.e., consumers, health professionals, payers and purchasers, etc.)*	*Poor.* No national priorities. Existing reviews do not address many patient populations (e.g., children, elderly) or the full continuum of services. Information on the comparative effectiveness of health services is largely lacking.	*Moderate to high.* Significant start up time required. Decision makers might have input into priority setting. Ability to respond depends on government oversight.	*High.* Actively seeks input from decision makers regarding priority topics for systematic reviews. Fewer procedural requirements/steps shorten response time.
Scientific rigor— *Methods minimize bias, are reliable, and completely reported*	*Poor.* Evidence-based methods may not be used; errors and poor documentation are common.	*Moderate to high.* Required by Program standards; program funding ensures that resources are available to support rigorous work. But performance will depend on well-trained staff with requisite scientific skills.	*Moderate to high.* Process maximizes likelihood that priority setting and systematic reviews would meet scientific standards. Reliance on disclosure of compliance with common standards and end user preference for guidelines produced according to standards.
Transparency— *Methods explicitly defined, consistently applied, and publicly available*	*Poor.* Appropriate documentation is often lacking. Information is often proprietary or not publicly available.	*High.* Required by Program standards and subject to federal disclosure requirements.	*Moderate to high.* Standards are publicly available. Reliance on disclosure of compliance with common standards and end user preference for guidelines produced according to standards.

Box 6-1. From a hypothetical perspective, a highly centralized effort (i.e., the agency model) appears to be more likely to offer maximum control over both evidence assessment and guideline development and, thus, theoretically a greater likelihood of optimizing the key principles. This model, however, is also likely to be the most costly, to generate more political opposition, and also to take more to time to establish than an approach that builds on current capacity. With the burgeoning array of new devices, medical technologies, and biological therapies, time is of the essence.

The critical difference between the hybrid Program infrastructure and the central agency model, are the entities that would formulate clinical guidelines. In both models, the quality of systematic reviews could be addressed through the application of rigorous process and reporting standards. The standards could be newly created or already developed standards that are endorsed by the Program. In the central agency model, the Program itself would oversee clinical guideline development as well as the systematic reviews. Under the hybrid approach, the Program would sponsor standards-based systematic reviews of high-priority topics by outside experts. In contrast with the agency model, the hybrid model assumes that existing independent entities—professional medical societies, payers, practice measurement groups, and others— would continue to develop clinical guidelines. The Program would actively encourage these organizations to voluntarily adopt Program standards for guideline development.

The agency and hybrid alternatives also differ with respect to the administrative infrastructure required to support the Program. Under the agency model, an extensive in-house staff would support or carry out key functions including priority setting, evidence reviews, and clinical guideline development. The hybrid approach would require fewer staff and build on current, outside capacity. The hybrid model also calls for an independent Priority Setting Advisory Committee, as described in Chapter 3, to establish and regularly update Program priorities for systematic review.

RECOMMENDATIONS FOR BUILDING THE PROGRAM INFRASTRUCTURE

This report has outlined an urgent imperative for immediate action to change how the nation marshals clinical evidence and applies it to identify the most effective clinical interventions. The nation's annual multibillion dollar investment in biomedical research and innovation has provided many important insights into human health and disease, yet only a fraction of one percent of U.S. spending on biomedical research is invested in identifying what constitutes sound and reliable evidence of the most effective health services (Emanuel et al., 2007). Evidence assessment (i.e., systematic review) is central to scientific inquiry into what is known and not known about what works in health care. The previous chapters outlined the committee's rationale and recommendations for three essential Program functions: priority setting, evidence assessment (systematic review), and developing standards for clinical guidelines. The following presents the committee's recommendations for establishing an infrastructure for organizing the three functions. The committee's complete set of recommendations are summarized in Box 6-2.

> Recommendation: Congress should direct the secretary of the U.S. Department of Health and Human Services to designate a single entity (the Program) with authority, overarching responsibility, sustained resources, and adequate capacity to ensure production of credible, unbiased information about what is known and not known about clinical effectiveness. The Program should
>
> - set priorities for, fund, and manage systematic reviews of clinical effectiveness and related topics;
> - develop a common language and standards for conducting systematic reviews of the evidence and for generating clinical guidelines and recommendations;
> - provide a forum for addressing conflicting guidelines and recommendations; and
> - prepare an annual report to Congress.

> Recommendation: The secretary of Health and Human Services should appoint a Clinical Effectiveness Advisory Board to oversee the Program. Its membership should be constituted to minimize bias due to conflict of interest and should include representation of diverse public and private sector expertise and interests.

> Recommendation: The Program should develop standards to minimize bias due to conflicts of interest for priority setting, evidence assessment, and recommendations development.

The committee urges that the Program incorporate substantial stakeholder involvement, develop (or endorse) methodologic and reporting standards for systematic reviews and clinical guidelines, and adopt rigorous standards for minimizing bias and conflict of interest in the Program.

An Independent Forum

Under the status quo, there are many conflicting clinical practice guidelines. Consumers, patients, health professionals, and others struggle to learn

---

BOX 6-2
Committee Recommendations

Building a Foundation (Chapter 6)

Congress should direct the secretary of the U.S. Department of Health and Human Services to designate a single entity (the Program) with authority, overarching responsibility, sustained resources, and adequate capacity to ensure production of credible, unbiased information about what is known and not known about clinical effectiveness. The Program should

- set priorities for, fund, and manage systematic reviews of clinical effectiveness and related topics;
- develop a common language and standards for conducting systematic reviews of the evidence and for generating clinical guidelines and recommendations;
- provide a forum for addressing conflicting guidelines and recommendations; and
- prepare an annual report to Congress.

The secretary of Health and Human Services should appoint a Clinical Effectiveness Advisory Board to oversee the Program. Its membership should be constituted to minimize bias due to conflict of interest and should include representation of diverse public and private sector expertise and interests.

The Program should develop standards to minimize bias due to conflicts of interest for priority setting, evidence assessment, and recommendations development.

Setting Priorities (Chapter 3)

The Program should appoint a standing Priority Setting Advisory Committee (PSAC) to identify high-priority topics for systematic reviews of clinical effectiveness.

- The priority setting process should be open, transparent, efficient, and timely.
- Priorities should reflect the potential for evidence-based practice to improve

---

which guideline is appropriate for which circumstances. The committee suggests that the Program sponsor ongoing, public meetings that are organized to help resolve differences between conflicting clinical guidelines and recommendations. Such an independent forum would provide an important public service.

Program Evaluation

The Program must be accountable to Congress and the public. The committee recommends that the Clinical Effectiveness Advisory Board health outcomes across the life span, reduce the burden of disease and health disparities, and eliminate undesirable variation.

- Priorities should also consider economic factors, such as the costs of treatment and the economic burden of disease.
- The membership of the PSAC should include a broad mix of expertise and interests and be chosen to minimize committee bias due to conflicts of interest.

Systematic Reviews (Chapter 4)

The Program should develop evidence-based, methodologic standards for systematic reviews, including a common language for characterizing the strength of evidence. The Program should fund reviewers only if they commit to and consistently meet these standards.

- The Program should invest in advancing the scientific methods underlying the conduct of systematic reviews and, when appropriate, update the standards for the reviews it funds.

The Program should assess the capacity of the research workforce to meet the Program's needs, and, if deemed appropriate, it should expand training opportunities in systematic review and comparative effectiveness research methods.

Developing Trusted Guidelines (Chapter 5)

Groups developing clinical guidelines or recommendations should use the Program's standards, document their adherence to the standards, and make this documentation publicly available.

To minimize bias due to conflicts of interest, panels should include a balance of competing interests and diverse stakeholders, publish conflict of interest disclosures, and prohibit voting by members with material conflicts.

Providers, public and private payers, purchasers, accrediting organizations, performance measurement groups, patients, consumers, and others should preferentially use clinical recommendations developed according to the Program standards

routinely evaluate the Program to ensure that it is fulfilling its purpose effectively and also submit an annual report on its activities and accomplishments to Congress.

UNANSWERED QUESTIONS

As Chapter 1 described, the scope of this study did not address several critical concerns that merit attention: where to place the Program and whether it should be public, private, or a public-private collaboration; program costs and sources of program funding; technical methods including the use of cost data and cost-effectiveness methods in assessing effectiveness; knowledge transfer and how to assure adherence to guidelines; how to reflect patient values and preferences in clinical guidelines; and legal issues.

REFERENCES

The AGREE Collaboration. 2001. *Appraisal of Guidelines for Research and Evaluation (AGREE) instrument.* http://www.agreecollaboration.org (accessed December 8, 2006).

AHRQ (Agency for Healthcare Research and Quality). 2007. *Effective Health Care—Home page* http://effectivehealthcare.ahrq.gov (accessed August 7, 2007).

America's Health Insurance Plans. 2007. *Setting a higher bar: We believe there is more the nation can do to improve quality and safety in health care.* Washington, DC: America's Health Insurance Plans.

Anderson, G. F., P. S. Hussey, B. K. Frogner, and H. R. Waters. 2005. Health spending in the United States and the rest of the industrialized world. *Health Affairs* 24(4):903-914.

Australian Safety & Efficacy Register of New Interventional Procedures–Surgical. 2005. *Annual Report.* Melbourne, Australia: Royal Australian College of Surgeons.

Battista, R. N. 2006. Expanding the scientific basis of health technology assessment: A research agenda for the next decade. *International Journal of Technology Assessment in Health Care* 22(3):275-280.

BCBSA (Blue Cross and Blue Shield Association). 2007a. *Blue Cross and Blue Shield Association's Technology Evaluation Center* http://www.bcbs.com/tec/index.html (accessed January 18, 2007).

————. 2007b. *Blue Cross and Blue Shield Association proposes payer-funded institute to evaluate what medical treatments work best* http://www.bcbs.com/news/bcbsa/blue-cross-and-blue-shield-association-proposes-payer-funded-institute.html (accessed May 2007).

Bhandari, M., F. Morrow, A. V. Kulkarni, and P. Tornetta. 2001. Meta-analyses in orthopaedic surgery: A systematic review of their methodologies. *Journal of Bone and Joint Surgery* 83A:15-24.

CADTH (Canadian Agency for Drugs and Technologies in Health). 2006. *Health technology assessment* http://www.cadth.ca/index.php/en/hta/ (accessed March 28, 2007).

Canadian Task Force on Preventive Health Care. 2005. *Evidence-based clinical prevention* http://www.ctfphc.org (accessed March 28, 2007).

Cochrane Collaboration. 2007. *The Cochrane Collaboration: The reliable source of evidence in health care* http://www.cochrane.org (accessed January 18, 2007).

Congressional Budget Office. 2007. Research on the comparative effectiveness of medical treatments: Options for an expanded federal role. *Testimony by Director Peter R. Orszag before House Ways and Means Subcommittee on Health* http://www.cbo.gov/ftpdocs/82xx/doc8209/Comparative_Testimony.pdf (accessed June 12, 2007).

Delaney, A., S. M. Bagshaw, A. Ferland, B. Manns, and K. B. Laupland. 2005. A systematic evaluation of the quality of meta-analyses in the critical care literature. *Critical Care* 9: R575-R582.

Department on Health and Ageing. 2006. *About us: Our role* http://www.health.gov.au/internet/wcms/publishing.nsf/Content/health-overview.htm (accessed March 28, 2007).

Draborg, E., and D. Gyrd-Hansen. 2005. Time-trends in health technology assessments: An analysis of developments in composition of international health technology assessments from 1989 to 2002. *International Journal of Technology Assessment in Health Care* 21(4):492-498.

ECRI. 2006. *About ECRI* http://www.ecri.org/About_ECRI/About_ECRI.aspx (accessed January 31, 2007).

Emanuel, E. J., V. R. Fuchs, and A. M. Garber. 2007. Essential elements of a technology and outcomes assessment initiative. *JAMA* 298(11):1323-1325.

García-Altés, A., S. Ondategui-Parra, and P. J. Neumann. 2004. Cross-national comparison of technology assessment processes. *International Journal of Technology Assessment in Health Care* 20(3):300-310.

Glenny, A. M., M. Esposito, P. Coulthard, and H. V. Worthington. 2003. The assessment of systematic reviews in dentistry. *European Journal of Oral Sciences* 111:85-92.

Gøtzsche, P. C., A. Hrobjartsson, K. Maric, and B. Tendal. 2007. Data extraction errors in meta-analyses that use standardized mean differences. *JAMA* 298(4):430-437.

GRADE Working Group. 2004. Grading quality of evidence and strength of recommendations. *BMJ* 328(7454):1490.

Gray, B. H. 1992. The legislative battle over health services research. *Health Affairs* 11(4): 38-66.

Gray, B. H., M. K. Gusmano, and S. Collins. 2003. AHCPR and the changing politics of health services research. *Health Affairs* w3.283.

Haute Autorité de Santé. 2007. *About HAS* http://www.has-sante.fr/portail/display.jsp?id=c_5443&pcid=c_5443 (accessed March 28, 2007).

Hayden, J. A., P. Cote, and C. Bombardier. 2006. Evaluation of the quality of prognosis studies in systematic reviews *Annals of Internal Medicine* 144:427-437.

Hayes, W. S. 2006. *Healthcare policy: Applying the evidence (PowerPoint presentation to the IOM HECS Committee meeting, November 7, 2006).* Washington, DC.

Higgins, J. T., and S. Green. 2006. *Cochrane handbook for systematic reviews of interventions 4.2.6 [updated September 2006],* The Cochrane Library, Issue 4, 2006. Chichester, UK: John Wiley & Sons, Ltd.

Institute for Quality and Efficiency in Health Care. 2007. *About us* http://www.iqwig.de/about-us.21.en.html (accessed March 28, 2007).

IOM (Institute of Medicine). 1992. *Setting priorities for health technologies assessment: A model process.* Edited by Donaldson, M. S., and H. C. Sox. Washington, DC: National Academy Press.

———. 1995. *Setting priorities for clinical practice guidelines.* Edited by Field, M. J. Washington, DC: National Academy Press.

———. 2001. *Crossing the quality chasm: A new health system for the 21st Century.* Washington, DC: National Academy Press.

———. 2007. *Learning what works best: The nation's need for evidence on comparative effectiveness in health care* http://www.iom.edu/ebm-effectiveness (accessed April 2007).

Jadad, A. R., and H. J. McQuay. 1996. Meta-analyses to evaluate analgesic interventions: A systematic qualitative review of their methodology. *Journal of Clinical Epidemiology* 49:235-243.

Jadad, A. R., M. Moher, G. P. Browman, L. Booker, C. Sigouin, M. Fuentes, and R. Stevens. 2000. Systematic reviews and meta-analyses on treatment of asthma: Critical evaluation. *BMJ* 320:537-540.

Jonsson, E. 2002. Development of health technology assessment in Europe. *International Journal of Technology Assessment in Health Care* 18(2):171-183.

Kristensen, F. B., and the EUnetHTA Partners. 2006. EUnetHTA and health policy-making in Europe. *Eurohealth* 12(1).

Kupersmith, J., N. Sung, M. Genel, H. Slavkin, R. Califf, R. Bonow, L. Sherwood, N. Reame, V. Catanese, C. Baase, J. Feussner, A. Dobs, H. Tilson, and E. A. Reece. 2005. Creating a new structure for research on health care effectiveness. *Journal of Investigative Medicine* 53(2):67-72.

Lexchin, J., L. A. Bero, B. Djulbegovic, and O. Clark. 2003. Pharmaceutical industry sponsorship and research outcome and quality: Systematic review. *BMJ* 326:1167-1170.

Lopert, R. 2006 (unpublished). *Pharmacoeconomics and drug subsidy in Australia—an account of the Australian approach.*

Mallen, C., G. Peat, and P. Croft. 2006. Quality assessment of observational studies is not commonplace in systematic reviews. *Journal of Clinical Epidemiology* 59:765-769.

Medicare Payment Advisory Commission. 2007. Chapter 2: Producing comparative effectiveness information. In *Report to the Congress: Promoting greater efficiency in Medicare* http://www.medpac.gov/documents/Jun07_EntireReport.pdf (accessed June 2007).

Miller, W. 2006. *Value-based coverage policy in the U.S. and UK: Different paths to a common goal.* Washington, DC: National Health Policy Forum.

Moher, D., D. J. Cook, S. Eastwood, I. Olkin, D. Rennie, D. F. Stroup, and the QUOROM Group. 1999. Improving the quality of reports of meta-analyses of randomized controlled trials: The QUOROM statement. *Lancet* 354:1896-1900.

Moher, D., J. Tetzlaff, A. C. Tricco, M. Sampson, and D. G. Altman. 2007. Epidemiology and reporting characteristics of systematic reviews. *PLoS Medicine* 4(3):447-455.

National Board of Health. 2007. *Danish Centre for Health Technology Assessment* http://www.sst.dk/Planlaegning_og_behandling/Medicinsk_teknologivurdering.aspx?lang=en (accessed March 28, 2007).

National Health and Medical Research Council. 2006. *Role of the NHMRC* http://www.nhmrc.gov.au/about/role/index.htm (accessed March 28, 2007).

National Research Council. 2004. *Eliminating health disparities: Measurement and data needs.* Edited by Ver Ploeg, M., and E. Perrin. Washington, DC: The National Academies Press.

NICE (National Institute for Health and Clinical Excellence). 2007. *About technology appraisals* http://www.nice.org.uk/page.aspx?o=202425 (accessed March 28, 2007).

NQF (National Quality Forum). 2006. *Organizational values* http://qualityforum.org/about/values.asp (accessed August 6, 2007).

Oliver, A., E. Mossialos, and R. Robinson. 2004. Health technology assessment and its influence on health-care priority setting. *International Journal of Technology Assessment in Health Care* 20(1):1-10.

Packer, C., S. Simpson, and A. Stevens (on behalf of EuroScan: the European Information Network on New and Changing Health Technologies). 2006. International diffusion of new health technologies: A ten-country analysis of six health technologies. *International Journal of Technology Assessment in Health Care* 22(4):419-428.

Sanders, J. M. 2002. Challenges, choices and Canada. *International Journal of Technology Assessment in Health Care* 18(2):199-202.

Shojania, K. G., M. Sampson, M. T. Ansari, J. Ji, S. Doucette, and D. Moher. 2007. How quickly do systematic reviews go out of date? A survival analysis. *Annals of Internal Medicine* 147:224-233.

Shortell, S. M., T. G. Rundall, and J. Hsu. 2007. Improving patient care by linking evidence-based medicine and evidence-based management. *JAMA* 298(6):673-676.

SIGN (Scottish Intercollegiate Guidelines Network). 2007. *Guideline Development Programme* http://www.sign.ac.uk/guidelines/development/index.html (accessed March 28, 2007).

Simpson, L. 2004. Lost in translation? Reflections on the role of research in improving health care for children. *Health Affairs* 23(5):125-130.

Steinberg, E. P., and B. R. Luce. 2005. Evidence based? Caveat emptor! *Health Affairs* 24(1):80-92.

Stroup, D. F., J. A. Berlin, S. C. Morton, I. Olkin, G. D. Williamson, D. Rennie, D. Moher, B. J. Becker, T. A. Sipe, and S. B. Thacker for the Meta-analysis Of Observational Studies in Epidemiology (MOOSE) Group. 2000. Meta-analysis of observational studies in epidemiology: A proposal for reporting. *JAMA* 283(15):2008-2012.

Velasco-Garrido, M., and R. Busse. 2005. *Health technology assessment: An introduction to objectives, role of evidence, and structure in Europe.* Brussels, Belgium: WHO European Observatory on Health Systems and Policies.

Whiting, P., A. W. Rutjes, J. Dinnes, J. B. Reitsma, P. M. Bossuyt, and J. Kleijnen. 2005. A systematic review finds that diagnostic reviews fail to incorporate quality despite available tools. *Journal of Clinical Epidemiology* 58:1-12.

Wilensky, G. R. 2006. Developing a center for comparative effectiveness information. *Health Affairs* w572.

Appendix A

Acronyms and Abbreviations

ACC	American College of Cardiology
ACP	American College of Physicians
ADA	American Dietetic Association
AGREE	Appraisal of Guidelines Research and Evaluation
AHA	American Heart Association
AHCPR	Agency for Health Care Policy and Research
AHRQ	Agency for Healthcare Research and Quality
AMA	American Medical Association
ASCO	American Society of Clinical Oncology
BCBSA	Blue Cross and Blue Shield Association
CADTH	Canadian Agency for Drugs and Technologies in Health
CDC	Centers for Disease Control and Prevention
CDER	Center for Drug Evaluation and Research
CEA	cost-effectiveness analysis
CMS	Centers for Medicare & Medicaid Services
COGS	Conference on Guideline Standardization
CONSORT	Consolidated Standards for Reporting Trials
DERP	Drug Effectiveness Review Project
EC	European Community
EPC	Evidence-based Practice Center
EUnetHTA	European Network for Health Technology Assessment
FDA	U.S. Food and Drug Administration
FDG	fluorodeoxyglucose
GDP	gross domestic product

HDC/ABMT	high dose chemotherapy with autologous bone marrow transplantation
HHS	U.S. Department of Health and Human Services
HTA	Health Technology Assessment
ICMJE	International Committee of Medical Journal Editors
IOM	Institute of Medicine
LILACS	Latin American Caribbean Health Sciences Literature
MCAC	Medicare Coverage Advisory Committee
MedCAC	Medicare Evidence Development and Coverage Advisory Committee
MOOSE	Meta-analysis Of Observational Studies in Epidemiology
MSAC	Medical Services Advisory Committee
NCQA	National Committee for Quality Assurance
NGC	National Guideline Clearinghouse
NHLBI	National Heart, Lung, and Blood Institute
NHS	National Health Service
NICE	National Institute for Health and Clinical Excellence
NIH	National Institutes of Health
NQF	National Quality Forum
OMAR	Office of Medical Applications of Research
OTA	U.S. Office of Technology Assessment
PET	positron emission tomography
PhRMA	Pharmaceutical Research and Manufacturers of America
PICO	population, intervention, comparison, and outcomes
PSAC	Priority Setting Advisory Committee
QUOROM	Quality of Reporting of Meta-analyses
RCT	randomized controlled trial
RWJF	Robert Wood Johnson Foundation
SAMHSA	Substance Abuse and Mental Health Services Administration
SIGN	Scottish Intercollegiate Guidelines Network
STARD	Standards for Reporting of Diagnostic Accuracy
STROBE	Strengthening the Reporting of Observational Studies in Epidemiology
TEC	Blue Cross and Blue Shield Association Technology Evaluation Center
USPSTF	U.S. Preventive Services Task Force
VA	Veterans Administration
VHA	Veterans Health Administration
WHO	World Health Organization

Appendix B

Workshop Agendas and Questions to Panelists

AGENDA—WORKSHOP 1

INSTITUTE OF MEDICINE

COMMITTEE ON REVIEWING EVIDENCE TO IDENTIFY
HIGHLY EFFECTIVE CLINICAL SERVICES

NOVEMBER 7, 2006

National Academy of Sciences Building
2101 Constitution Avenue, NW, Lecture Room, Washington, DC

Workshop Objective: To review three case studies that reveal the challenges that decision makers face when trying to determine the clinical effectiveness of healthcare technologies.

8:30   Welcome and introductory remarks—*Barbara McNeil, Chair, Institute of Medicine (IOM) Committee*

8:45   Panel 1—PET Scan for Alzheimer's Disease. Moderator: Dick Justman (UnitedHealthcare)
        Marilyn Albert, Johns Hopkins University School of Medicine, Division of Cognitive Neuroscience
        David Matchar, Duke University Medical School, Center for Clinical Health Policy Research

Sean Tunis, Center for Medical Technology Policy
Susan Molchan, Alzheimer's Disease Neuroimaging Initiative, National Institute on Aging (NIH)

Question & Answer/Open Discussion

10:15   Break

10:30   **Panel 2—Avastin and Lucentis for Age Related Macular Degeneration. Moderator: Diana Petitti (Kaiser Permanente, Southern California)**
Reginald Sanders, American Society of Retina Specialists
Winifred Hayes, Hayes, Inc.
Steve Phurrough, CMS Coverage and Analysis Group
Dan Martin, Emory University School of Medicine

Question & Answer/Open Discussion

12:15   Lunch

1:00   **Panel 3—Screening and Treating Colorectal Cancer—The Fecal DNA Test and an Assay for Irinotecan Toxicity. Moderator: Steve Shak (Genomic Health, Inc.)**
Barry Berger, Exact Sciences Corporation
Margaret Piper, Blue Cross and Blue Shield Association Technology Evaluation Center
Richard Goldberg, University of North Carolina, Chapel Hill
Atiqur Rahman, Food and Drug Administration, Center for Drug Evaluation and Research

Question & Answer/Open Discussion

3:00   Break

3:15   **Panel 4—Experts React. Moderator: Hal Sox, Vice Chair, IOM Committee**
Daniel Cain, Cain Brothers
Peter Juhn, Health Policy and Evidence, Johnson & Johnson
Cindy Mulrow, University of Texas and the American College of Physicians
David Ransohoff, University of North Carolina Chapel Hill, School of Medicine
Earl Steinberg, Resolution Health

5:00   **Adjourn**

Questions for the Panelists—Workshop 1
November 7, 2006

Panel 1—PET Scans for Alzheimer's

- What does this experience show about the feasibility of coverage with evidence development under Medicare?
- What roles did evidence assessment and political pressure have in this coverage decision? How is this experience instructive for future cases?
- What challenges were involved in ensuring that the evidence available on PET was applicable to everyday clinical practice?

Panel 2—Lucentis/Avastin

- Was the substantial uptake in Avastin use for wet AMD justifiable given the lack of evidence and the needs of the patient population?
- How do evidence reviewers and payers address the relative effectiveness of Lucentis and Avastin given the limited data?
- Given the state of the evidence base, what role should cost play in payer decisions?
- What does this case study say about the societal need for more clinical data and information and the mechanisms by which data development is financed?
- How will the head-to-head trial supported by NIH alter their role in terms of assessing cost effectiveness?

Panel 3—Genetic Tests

- Do you think that more of these types of tests will be developed [toxicity, and non-invasive screening]? How will experiences with these technologies affect the development of more similar tests?
- Are non-invasive screenings (genetic byproduct screening) and toxicity testing the "wave(s) of the future"? What types or levels of evidence are needed to recommend replacement of current therapies? Will comparative testing be done as newer technologies emerge?
- Are there specific challenges due to the nature of the populations qualified for testing? (Such as, are the populations so small as to affect the feasibility of large clinical trials?)
- As the evidence for these tests is emerging, how do gaps in evidence compare with more traditional technologies?

- What are the labeling issues for these technologies? What needs to be included and what would prompt a change?
- Is patient compliance and invasiveness considered when determining effectiveness?

Panel 4—Reactor

- What role did evidence play in these examples (as compared to other influences such as political pressure and provider experience)?
- Was the process of data collection and assessment able to keep pace with consumer and provider demand?
- In what ways did lack of data influence the process?
- What is the likelihood that the gaps in data will be filled (and in a timely manner)?
- How should current standards and methods in evidence assessment change in this era of personalized medicine, new biologic therapies, and advanced imaging techniques (if at all)?
- What needs to change to expedite the introduction of clinical services that are potentially highly effective (e.g., expediting the clinical trial process, and obtaining different funding mechanisms for investigations).
- How might information about new technologies be made more accessible for patients?

AGENDA—WORKSHOP 2

INSTITUTE OF MEDICINE

COMMITTEE ON REVIEWING EVIDENCE TO IDENTIFY
HIGHLY EFFECTIVE CLINICAL SERVICES

JANUARY 25, 2007

National Academy of Sciences Building
2101 Constitution Avenue, NW, Lecture Room, Washington, DC

8:30   **Welcome and introductory remarks**—*Barbara McNeil, Chair,
Institute of Medicine Committee*

8:35   **Panel 1—Using Systematic Reviews to Develop Clinical
Recommendations. Moderator: Richard Marshall**
Carolyn Clancy, Agency for Healthcare Research and Quality
Mary Barton, U.S. Preventive Services Task Force

Steven Findlay, Consumers Union
Ray Gibbons, American Heart Association

Question & Answer/Open Discussion

9:55 **Panel 2—Using Systematic Reviews to Develop Quality Measures and Practice Standards. Moderator: Lisa Simpson**
Janet Corrigan, National Quality Forum
Greg Pawlson, National Committee for Quality Assurance
Dennis O'Leary, Joint Commission on Accreditation of
  Healthcare Organizations
Cary Sennett, AMA-convened Physician Consortium for
  Performance Improvement

Question & Answer/Open Discussion

11:15 **Panel 3—Approaches to Priority Setting: Identifying Topics and Selection Criteria. Moderator: Dana Goldman**
Richard Justman, UnitedHealthcare
Kay Dickersin, Cochrane USA
Jean Slutsky, AHRQ Effective Health Care Program
Naomi Aronson, BCBSA Technology Evaluation Center

Question & Answer/Open Discussion

12:30 **Lunch**

1:00 **Panel 4—Stakeholders Forum. Moderator: Robert Galvin**
Kathy Buto, Johnson & Johnson
Art Small, Genentech
Vivian Coates, ECRI
Jim Weinstein, Dartmouth-Hitchcock Medical Center

Question & Answer/Open Discussion

INSTITUTE OF MEDICINE WORKSHOP

REVIEWING EVIDENCE TO IDENTIFY HIGHLY EFFECTIVE CLINICAL SERVICES

JANUARY 25, 2007

PANEL 1—USING SYSTEMATIC REVIEWS TO DEVELOP
CLINICAL RECOMMENDATIONS

Moderator: Richard Marshall (Harvard Vanguard Medical Associates)
Panelists: Carolyn Clancy (AHRQ), Mary Barton (USPSTF), Steven
             Findlay (Consumers Union), and Ray Gibbons (American
             Heart Association)

*The objective of this panel discussion is to learn about the experiences of
well-regarded organizations that use systematic reviews or other syntheses
of bodies of evidence to develop clinical recommendations. AHRQ serves
multiple roles; generator of evidence (e.g., DEcIDE, CERTS), synthesizer
of evidence (e.g., Evidence-based Practice Center Program), and developer
of clinical recommendations (e.g., USPSTF). The USPSTF assesses and synthesizes the evidence on preventive services and issues clinical recommendations based on these bodies of evidence. Consumers Union's Best Buy Drugs
Program relies on evidence-based analyses of the safety and effectiveness of
prescription drugs to help consumers choose the drug best suited to their
medical needs. The American Heart Association (in collaboration with the
American College of Cardiology) synthesizes bodies of evidence on selected
topics and draws from other reviews to develop clinical practice guidelines
for cardiovascular care.*

Questions for the Panelists

1. Who is the principal audience for your clinical recommendations?
    Have you assessed their use of the recommendations? Approximately
    how often does your audience follow your clinical recommendations:

    • In full, _____ percent
    • In part, _____ percent

2. How do you identify and prioritize areas for which clinical
    recommendations are necessary?

3. How do you identify sources of evidence on clinical effectiveness?
    Which criteria (if any) do you use to judge quality of evidence?

4. How would you characterize the available evidence on the clinical

questions you address? Does it sufficiently cover services and populations of interest? What are the critical gaps (if any)?

5. Do you incorporate observational and other nonrandomized data in your evidence syntheses? If yes, what are the parameters for their use?

6. How do you respond to pressing demands for clinical recommendations when the body of evidence is insufficient or when the available evidence is relevant to only a subset of patients? Approximately how often do you make recommendations in the absence of sufficient data in these cases?

7. What resources does your organization dedicate to developing evidence-based clinical recommendations (e.g., staff time, special committee responsibility, conferences)?

INSTITUTE OF MEDICINE WORKSHOP

REVIEWING EVIDENCE TO IDENTIFY HIGHLY EFFECTIVE CLINICAL SERVICES

JANUARY 25, 2007

PANEL 2—USING SYSTEMATIC REVIEWS TO DEVELOP
QUALITY MEASURES AND PRACTICE STANDARDS

Moderator: Lisa Simpson (Cincinnati Children's Hospital Medical Center)

Panelists: Janet Corrigan (NQF), Greg Pawlson (NCQA), Dennis O'Leary (JCAHO), Cary Sennett (AMA-convened Physician Consortium)

The objective of this panel discussion is to learn about the experiences of leading organizations that are at the forefront of U.S. efforts to develop, implement, and improve evidence-based clinical practice standards. The mission of the NQF is to promote quality improvement in healthcare by endorsing national performance measures. NCQA's HEDIS measures are used to assess health plan performance on various dimensions of care. JCAHO's ORYX initiative incorporates outcome performance measurement into the accreditation process for health care organizations. The AMA-convened Physician Consortium for Performance Improvement® (Consortium) has developed more than 100 performance measures for practicing physicians. The Consortium includes more than 100 medical specialty and state medical societies, the Council of Medical Specialty Societies, American Board of Medical Specialties and its member-boards, experts in methodology and data collection, the Agency for Healthcare Research and Quality, and the Centers for Medicare & Medicaid Services.

Questions for the Panelists

1. How do you identify areas for which quality measures or practice standards are necessary?

2. Who is the principal audience for your evidence-based measures/ standards? What factors promote your credibility and establish you as a trusted source of information for these groups?

3. How do you respond to pressing demands for measures/standards when the relevant body of evidence is insufficient? Approximately how often do you make recommendations in the absence of sufficient data in these cases?

4. Do you have a mechanism for influencing research to produce needed evidence? What are your thoughts about the emerging practice of coverage with evidence development?

5. How would you characterize the available evidence on the clinical questions you address? Does it sufficiently cover services and populations of interest? What are the critical gaps (if any)?

6. Do you consider observational and other nonrandomized data on clinical effectiveness? If yes, what are the parameters for their use?

7. What resources does your organization use to identify, assess, and incorporate evidence syntheses in your clinical quality measures/ standards (e.g., staff time, special committee responsibility, conferences)?

INSTITUTE OF MEDICINE WORKSHOP

REVIEWING EVIDENCE TO IDENTIFY HIGHLY EFFECTIVE CLINICAL SERVICES

JANUARY 25, 2007

PANEL 3—APPROACHES TO PRIORITY SETTING:
IDENTIFYING TOPICS AND SELECTION

Moderator: Dana Goldman
Panelists: Richard Justman (UnitedHealthcare), Kay Dickersin

(Cochrane USA), Jean Slutsky (AHRQ Effective Health Care Program), Naomi Aronson (BCBSA TEC)

The objective of this panel discussion is to learn how these leading organizations prioritize their efforts to conduct systematic reviews on clinical effectiveness. UnitedHealthcare is one of the nation's largest health plans with an estimated 22 million covered lives. The Cochrane Collaboration is an international, not-for-profit organization that produces and disseminates systematic reviews of health care interventions. AHRQ's Effective Health Care Program is the leading federal agency charged with systematically reviewing and synthesizing evidence on clinical effectiveness. BCBSA TEC, an AHRQ-designated Evidence-based Practice Center, is a highly respected source of evidence-based assessments of the clinical effectiveness of medical procedures, devices, and drugs.

Questions for the Panelists

1. How do you identify topics? Please provide a detailed outline of your approach, using, for example, last year's topics.

2. How would you characterize the yield from your efforts to identify topics? Does it capture a broad spectrum of services? What about surgical procedures? Existing services? Behavioral health? Disease management? Children's health?

3. What are your criteria for selecting topics and how are the criteria implemented (e.g., through a formal process and quantitative method)?

4. Do you have a mechanism for picking up missed but important topics? How often (in retrospect) has your horizon scanning failed to identify a key service? Consider the past two years in answering this question.

5. How do you rank priorities? Please be specific as to the criteria used. How many of the priority topics are addressed each year?

6. What factors, if any, can override already determined priorities?

7. Has this approach worked well given your objectives? What are the strengths and weaknesses of the process?

8. What resources are involved in this activity (e.g., staff time, special committee responsibility, conferences)?

INSTITUTE OF MEDICINE WORKSHOP

REVIEWING EVIDENCE TO IDENTIFY HIGHLY EFFECTIVE CLINICAL SERVICES

JANUARY 25, 2007

PANEL 4—STAKEHOLDERS FORUM

Moderator: Robert Galvin (General Electric)
Panelists: Kathy Buto (J&J), Vivian Coates (ECRI), Art Small
(Genentech), James Weinstein (Dept. of Orthopedics,
Dartmouth-Hitchcock Medical Center)

The objective of this panel discussion is to learn key stakeholders' views on how highly effective clinical services are identified. Johnson & Johnson is one of the world's largest manufacturers of medical devices, drugs, and equipment. ECRI, an AHRQ-designated Evidence-based Practice Center, is a highly respected source of evidence-based assessments of the clinical effectiveness of medical procedures, devices, and drugs. Genentech is one of the world's leading biotech companies. Dartmouth-Hitchcock's department of orthopedics is the primary site of a 5-year, $14 million trial comparing surgical to nonsurgical treatments for certain back problems.

Questions for the Panelists

This IOM Committee has been charged with recommending an approach to identifying highly effective clinical services across the spectrum of care— from prevention, diagnosis, treatment, and rehabilitation, to end-of-life care and palliation. In light of this charge and from the perspective of your organization, please answer the following:

1. How do you think that priorities should be set for services that need evidence development or synthesis?

2. What is your organization's current role in the development, use, and analysis of evidence on the clinical effectiveness of health care services (including drugs, devices, procedures, and other methods used to promote health or rehabilitation)?

3. Several groups and individuals—perhaps most recently Gail Wilensky in a *Health Affairs* piece[1]—have proposed the establishment of a sizable entity to effect a quantum leap in the national capacity to assess the comparative effectiveness of health care services. How

---

[1]Wilensky G. 2006. *Health Affairs Web Exclusive* w572-w585. Bethesda, MD: Project Hope.

might such a venture provide benefits, what would be the key concerns, and what would be the implications for your organization?

4. The U.S. Preventive Services Task Force evaluates evidence and develops recommendations for clinical preventive services.[2] How would your organization respond to the formation of a similar task force that provided the same function for clinical interventions, e.g., diagnostic testing, treatment, etc?

---

[2]Harris, R. P., M. Helfand, S. H. Woolf, K. N. Lohr, C. D. Mulrow, S. M. Teutsch, and D. Atkins. 2001. Current methods of the U.S. Preventive Services Task Force: A review of the process. *American Journal of Preventive Medicine* 20(3 Suppl):21-35.

Appendix C

Template for Submissions of Topics to the Agency for Healthcare Research and Quality

Appendix
Template for Submissions of Topics
for AHRQ Evidence Reports or Technology Assessments

Please complete the following information to nominate an AHRQ evidence report or technology assessment topic. Topic nominations should be submitted to Acting Director, Evidence-based Practice Centers (EPC) Program, Center for Outcomes and Evidence at AHRQ. Please e-mail this document to epc@ahrq.gov.

AHRQ will evaluate nominations based on: (a) the rationale and evidence of the importance of the topic; (b) plans for rapid translation of the resulting EPC report findings; (c) plans for dissemination of derivative products; and (d) plans for measuring the use and impact of an EPC report.

Note: Please refer to the Federal Register Notice (http://edocket.access.gpo.gov/2005/04-27058.htm) for the due date of this topic nomination; topic nominations are typically due 50-60 days following the publication of the Federal Register Notice, for submittal of topics for consideration in the current fiscal year. However, topic nominations also can be submitted electronically to AHRQ on an ongoing basis.

Nominating Organization Information

Please provide contact information and an overview of the nominating organization, such as its mission, priorities, research agenda and/or interest or commitment to evidence analyses, etc.

Organization Name:	
Contact Name: Title:	
Address:	
Phone: **E-mail:**	

Overview of Organization:

Proposed Evidence Assessment Topic and Evidence Questions

Please provide a **brief** description of the proposed topic. Appropriate topics are those that focus on clinical or behavioral issues or those that address organization, financing or delivery of health care.

Brief Name of Topic:

Please provide 3 to 5 *well-defined* evidence questions to guide the evidence review or technology assessment. (Additional well-defined evidence questions may be provided if necessary to address the topic.) An appropriate evidence question is one that can be addressed by a review of the available evidence by an EPC. Evidence questions should address, wherever applicable, particular indications, populations, interventions, care settings, and/or outcomes (e.g., effectiveness, safety, cost-effectiveness, etc.) of interest.

Example 1

> **INSTEAD OF:** What are the appropriate indications for [procedure X]?
>
> **TRY:** Does [procedure X] improve [certain outcomes] for [certain types of] patients? **OR** For what types of patients is there strong evidence that [procedure X] improves [certain outcomes]?

Example 2

> **INSTEAD OF:** What are the effects on health care of defined contribution models?
>
> **TRY:** How does utilization of previously covered health care services change when employers offer defined contribution models to their employees?

In developing your evidence questions, please consider the guidance on framing evidence questions for AHRQ Topic Nominations outlined in the Partners Guide (see page 10).

Evidence Question #1

Evidence Question #2

Evidence Question #3

Evidence Question #4

Evidence Question #5

Please complete the first box below for clinical and/or behavioral topics or the second box for organizational, financial and health care delivery topics.

Defined Condition and Target Population of the Intervention
(for clinical and/or behavioral topics)

Nomination of clinical and behavioral topics should focus on specific aspects of screening, prevention, diagnosis, treatment, rehabilitation of a particular disease or condition; alternative or complementary therapies; and/or on one or more procedures, interventions or other technologies used in the management of the disease or condition. Please provide below a description of the condition and/or disease and target population of the intervention to be assessed in the evidence review.

Defined Organizational/Financial Arrangement or Structure
(for organizational, finance and health care delivery topics)

Nominations of organization, financing and delivery topics should focus on specific aspects of the organization, financing or delivery of health care. Among the broad range of potential topics are such examples as risk-adjustment methodologies, market performance measures, provider payment methodologies, insurance purchasing tools, etc. Please provide below a description of the organizational/financial arrangement or structure to be assessed in the evidence review.

Topic Rationale and Supporting Evidence

Please provide a concise narrative justification for the topic to be nominated along with supporting evidence on the relevance and importance of the topic. This section is organized by key factors that will be considered in the selection of topics for AHRQ evidence reports and technology assessments. *Please provide information under each selection factor that is applicable to the topic.* It is not necessary to fill in each section.

Description of the burden of disease, including severity, incidence and/or prevalence or relevance of organizational/financial topic to the general population and/or AHRQ's priority populations (i.e., low-income groups, minority groups, women, children, elderly, individuals with special health care needs)

High costs associated with a condition, procedure, treatment, technology, organization/financial topic, taking into account the number of people needing such care, the unit cost of care and related or indirect costs

Impact potential of an evidence report on this topic to improve patient and/or provider decision-making, improve health outcomes and/or reduce costs

Availability of scientific and/or administrative data and bibliographies of studies on the topic to support the systematic review and analysis of the topic

References to significant differences in practice patterns or results of health outcomes, alternative therapies and/or related controversies or uncertainties about the topic

Relevance to the needs of the Medicare, Medicaid and other federal health care programs

Plans for Translation of the Evidence
Report into Derivative Products

EPCs take approximately one year to produce evidence reports/technology assessments. Organizations that nominate topics are responsible for translating the evidence reports and/or technology assessments into products that are useful for their memberships or other target groups. Please describe your plans for translating the evidence reports into quality improvement tools (e.g., clinical practice guidelines, performance measures), educational programs and/or coverage or reimbursement policies.

Plans for Dissemination of These Derivative
Products to its Membership

Organizations nominating topics are responsible for disseminating the derivative products to their memberships or other target groups, as appropriate. Please describe your organization's plans for disseminating these quality improvement tools (e.g., clinical practice guidelines, performance measures), educational programs, etc. Please include a description of the target groups of these products (e.g., organizational members, health professionals, patient/consumer groups, regulators, etc.), proposed dissemination media (e.g., journal articles, print media, Internet), and timeframe for dissemination.

How Organization will Measure Use of the
Products and Impact of Such Use

Organizations nominating topics are responsible for measuring the use of the derivative products and their impact. Please describe the process by which your organization will measure the use of the products and the impact of such use on clinical care. In addition, briefly describe any barriers to use or implementation of the derivative products (e.g., lack of funding, lack of patient compliance, professional resistance) and possible means to overcome these barriers (e.g., continuing education, changes in payment policies).

Appendix D

Standards for Reporting Meta-Analyses of Clinical Trials and Observational Studies: QUOROM and MOOSE

QUOROM CHECKLIST

Improving the quality of reports of meta-analyses of randomised controlled trials (RCTs): The QUOROM statement checklist

Heading	Subheading	Descriptor
Title		Identify the report as a meta-analysis [or systematic review] of RCTs
Abstract		Use a structured format
		Describe
	Objectives	The clinical question explicitly
	Data sources	The databases (i.e., list) and other information sources
	Review methods	The selection criteria (i.e., population, intervention, outcome, and study design); methods for validity assessment, data abstraction, and study characteristics, and quantitative data synthesis in sufficient detail to permit replication
	Results	Characteristics of the RCTs included and excluded; qualitative and quantitative findings (i.e., point estimates and confidence intervals); and subgroup analyses
	Conclusion	The main results
		Describe
Introduction		The explicit clinical problem, biological rationale for the intervention and rationale for review

Methods	Searching	The information sources, in detail (e.g., databases, registers, personal files, expert informants, agencies, hand-searching), and any restrictions (years considered, publication status, language of publication)
	Selection	The inclusion and exclusion criteria (defining population, intervention, principal outcomes, and study design)
	Validity assessment	The criteria and process used (e.g., masked conditions, quality assessment, and their findings)
	Data abstraction	The process or processes used (e.g., completed independently, in duplicate)
	Study characteristics	The type of study design, participants' characteristics, details of intervention, outcome definitions, &c, and how clinical heterogeneity was assessed
	Quantitative data Synthesis	The principal measures of effect (e.g., relative risk), method of combining results (statistical testing and confidence intervals), handling of missing data; how statistical heterogeneity was assessed; a rationale for any a-priori sensitivity and subgroup analyses; and any assessment of publication bias
Results	Trial flow	Provide a meta-analysis profile summarizing trial flow (see figure)
	Study characteristics	Present descriptive data for each trial (e.g., age, sample size, intervention, dose, duration, follow-up period)
	Quantitative data synthesis	Report agreement on the selection and validity assessment; present simple summary results (for each treatment group in each trial, for each primary outcome); present data needed to calculate effect sizes and confidence intervals in intention-to-treat analyses (e.g. 2×2 tables of counts, means and SDs (standard deviations), proportions)
Discussion		Summarize key findings; discuss clinical inferences based on internal and external validity; interpret the results in light of the totality of available evidence; describe potential biases in the review process (e.g., publication bias); and suggest a future research agenda

Quality of reporting of meta-analyses

Reprinted from *Lancet*, Vol 354, Moher, D., D. J. Cook, S. Eastwood, I. Olkin, D. Rennie, D. F. Stroup, and the QUOROM Group. Improving the quality of reports of meta-analyses of randomised controlled trials: The QUOROM statement, 1896-1900, Copyright 1999, with permission from Elsevier.

Improving the quality of reports of meta-analyses of randomized controlled trials: The QUOROM statement flow diagram

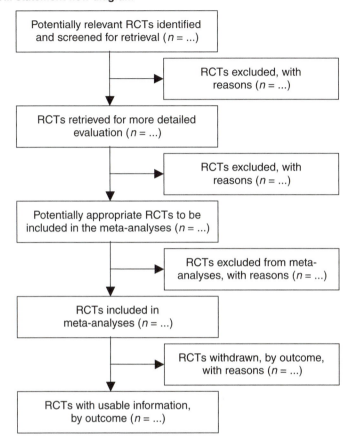

Reprinted from *Lancet*, Vol 354, Moher, D., D. J. Cook, S. Eastwood, I. Olkin, D. Rennie, D. F. Stroup, and the QUOROM Group. Improving the quality of reports of meta-analyses of randomised controlled trials: The QUOROM statement, 1896-1900, Copyright 1999, with permission from Elsevier.

NOTE: The QUOROM Statement is currently being updated under the name PRISMA (Preferred Reporting Items for Systematic Reviews and Meta-Analyses). PRISMA will include a 27-item checklist and four-phase flow diagram. The intent of the update is to reflect a more comprehensive understanding of conceptual issues, methodological advances, and practical innovations in the conduct and reporting of systematic reviews.

MOOSE CHECKLIST

A Proposed Reporting Checklist for Authors, Editors, and Reviews of Meta-analyses Of Observational Studies

---

Reporting of background should include
   Problem definition
   Hypothesis statement
   Description of study outcome(s)
   Type of exposure of intervention used
   Type of study designs used
   Study population
Reporting of search strategy should include
   Qualifications of searchers (e.g., librarians and investigators)
   Search strategy, including time period included in the synthesis and keywords
   Effort to include all available studies, including contact with authors
   Databases and registries searched
   Search software used, name and version, including special features used (eg, explosion)
   Use of hand searching (e.g., reference lists of obtained articles)
   List of citations located and those excluded, including justification
   Method of addressing articles published in languages other than English
   Method of handling abstracts and unpublished studies
   Description of any contact with authors
Reporting of methods should include
   Description of relevance or appropriateness of studies assembled for assessing the hypothesis to be tested
   Rationale for the selection and coding of data (e.g., sound clinical principles or convenience)
   Documentation of how data were classified and coded (e.g., multiple raters, blinding, and interrater reliability)
   Assessment of confounding (e.g., comparability of cases and controls in studies where appropriate)
   Assessment of study quality, including blinding of quality assessors; stratification or regression on possible predictors of study results
   Assessment of heterogeneity
   Description of statistical methods (e.g., complete description of fixed or random effects models, justification of whether the chosen models account for predictors of study results, dose-response models, or cumulative meta-analyses) in sufficient detail to be replicated
   Provision of appropriate tables and graphics
Reporting of results should include
   Graphic summarizing individual study estimates and overall estimate
   Table giving descriptive information for each study included
   Results of sensitivity testing (e.g., subgroup analysis)
   Indication of statistical uncertainty findings
Reporting of discussion should include
   Quantitative assessment of bias (e.g., publication bias)
   Justification for exclusion (e.g., exclusion of non-English-language citations)
   Assessment of quality of included studies
Reporting of conclusions include
   Consideration of alternative explanations for observed results

Generalization of the conclusions (i.e., appropriate for the data presented and within
  the domain of the literature review)
Guidelines for future research
Disclosure of funding source

Reprinted, with permission, from *JAMA* 2000, 283:2008-2012. Copyright 2000 by American Medical Association. All rights reserved.

REFERENCES

Cochrane Collaboration. 2006. Revising the QUOROM Statement. *Cochrane News* 37 http://www.cochrane.org/newslett/CochraneNews37lores.pdf (accessed September 12, 2007).
Moher, D., D. J. Cook, S. Eastwood, I. Olkin, D. Rennie, D. F. Stroup, and the QUOROM Group. 1999. Improving the quality of reports of meta-analyses of randomised controlled trials: The QUOROM statement. *Lancet* 354:1896-1900.
PLoS editors. 2007. Many reviews are systematic but some are more transparent and completely reported than others. *PLoS Medicine* 4(3):e147.
Stroup, D. F., J. A. Berlin, S. C. Morton, I. Olkin, G. D. Williamson, D. Rennie, D. Moher, B. J. Becker, T. A. Sipe, S. B. Thacker, and the Meta-analysis Of Observational Studies in Epidemiology (MOOSE) Group. 2000. Meta-analysis of observational studies in epidemiology: A proposal for reporting. *JAMA* 283(15):2008-2012.

Appendix E

Examples of ECRI Institute and Hayes, Inc., Quick Turnaround Reports

Efficacy of Human Papillomavirus (HPV) Vaccines for Prevention of Cervical Cancer[1]

Thank you for using ECRI's Health Technology Assessment Information Service (HTAIS). This Hotline Response provides information about **Efficacy of Human Papillomavirus (HPV) Vaccines for Prevention of Cervical Cancer**. To prepare this Hotline Response we consulted a number of information resources. We provide a description of these resources, including a complete outline of the databases we searched, our search strategies, and the search results at the end of this Response. ECRI has published a related Hotline (1); to access this and other materials on HPV, search the HTAIS Web site using the search term: *HPV*.

General Comments:

About Human Papillomavirus
The human papillomavirus (HPV) is a sexually transmitted virus carried by over half of the sexually active population in the United States. Prevalence estimates of HPV in the United States range from 6.2 million to 20

NOTE: These reports are provided as examples and are not intended to represent an endorsement by the committee.

---

[1]Reprinted, with permission, from *ECRI* 2006. Copyright 2007 by ECRI Institute.

million people. In most people, the infection is entirely asymptomatic and causes no disease. However, in some people, HPV can cause genital or anal warts, recurrent respiratory papillomatosis (RRP) lesions, and/or cancer, most notably of the cervix. Cervical cancer is the 11th most common cancer among US women, and the second most common cause of cancer in women worldwide. An estimated 9,710 new cases of cervical cancer will occur in the United States alone in 2006, and 3,700 women will die from it. Although the conditions it causes may be treatable, HPV infection has no treatment, and use of condoms may not prevent HPV transmission. (See Centers for Disease Control and Prevention (CDC) links in section 8 of the Search Summary) Other cancers thought to be caused by HPV include vaginal, vulvar, and head and neck cancer. Additional information on HPV and HPV-related diseases can be found through the Web sites listed in section 8 of the Search Summary.

About HPV Vaccines

Two major pharmaceutical companies have developed vaccines for HPV. These vaccines are administered in three injections: at day 1, month 2, and month 6. There are over 100 known strains of HPV, but only a few have been causally associated with cancer. Vaccines are intended to protect against the most dangerous strains of HPV. The following paragraphs include details from an Advisory Committee on Immunization Practices meeting held at the CDC in February 2006 regarding these vaccines. (See link in section 8 of the Search Summary)

GlaxoSmithKline has produced a recombinant vaccine (Cervarix) against HPV strains 16 and 18, which are the strains responsible for 70% of cases of cervical cancer. This vaccine has been tested in 1,113 women for over two years. It was found to be well tolerated, with minimal, minor adverse events. It was also found to be highly efficacious, with 100% protection against persistent HPV (meaning the infection has not resolved within six months and is therefore more likely to lead to pathological changes) caused by the target strains. Through the follow-up period, 93% of patients had normal pap smears. 53 months after vaccination, 98% of patients still had HPV antigens thought to be protective. Phase III studies enrolling more than 30,000 patients internationally are currently underway.

Merck & Co. has developed a vaccine (Gardasil) against HPV strains 16 and 18, as well as strains 6 and 11. Together, these strains account for more than 90% of cases of genital warts and RRP, in addition to protecting against cervical cancer. This vaccine has also been studied in men, who can develop cancer, RRP, and genital warts from HPV. In addition, men can transmit the virus to women, potentially causing cervical cancer in their partners. The clinical trial for this vaccine enrolled 27,000 women and children in four continents. Thus far, results have been analyzed for 20,541 recipients, and 100% prophylactic efficacy has been found for cervical, vaginal, and vulvar cancers caused by HPT strains 16 and 18. It was also found to be efficacious in preventing re-infection in women who had previously been infected with HPV. Reported serious (unspecified) adverse events were low, affecting 0.4% of 27,000 women.

The US Food and Drug Administration advisory panel on Vaccines and Related Biological Products has recommended approval of Merck & Co.'s application to market Gardasil. Formal approval by the FDA was received on June 8, 2006. Documents presented to the committee and final approval documents can be viewed through the Web sites listed in section 6 of the Search Summary.

Recent Clinical Literature

Our searches identified 14 randomized, controlled trials (RCTs), 37 traditional reviews, and 3 cost analyses. These publications are categorized in Table 1. We subdivided the RCTs by clinical outcomes (e.g. persistent infection and other treatment-requiring conditions) and intermediate outcomes (e.g. antibody titers). Since clinical outcomes are of more importance in healthcare, we summarized findings for these RCTs in Table 2. Although no evidence-based conclusions can be drawn from abstracts, the results appear promising. The three cost analyses found that vaccinating for HPV should be less costly than frequently screening for its effects (i.e. administering pap smears annually rather than tri-annually) and treating its sequelae (i.e. repeated pap smears, colposcopy, LEEP (loop electrosurgical excision procedure) for dysplasia, and cancer treatments).

Table 1. Recent Clinical Literature

Publication Type		Number of Identified Publications	References
Randomized, Controlled Trials (RCTs)	Clinical Outcomes	4	2-5
	Intermediate Outcomes	10	6-15
Reviews		37	16-52
Cost Analyses		3	53-55

Table 2. Randomized, Controlled Trials on Vaccine Efficacy in Clinical Outcomes

Citation	Vaccine Studied	Population	Follow-Up Time	Findings
Harper et al. 2006 (2)	Strains 16 and 18 (n=393) and placebo (n=383)	Adult women	4.5 years	Efficacy of vaccine against: • incident infection was 96.9% (95% CI 81.3-99.0%) • persistent infection at 1yr was 100% (95% CI 33.6-100%) • cervical intraepithelial neoplasia was 100% (95% CI 42.4-100%)
Mao et al. 2006 (3)	Strain 16 (n=755) or placebo (n=750)	Women aged 16-23 years	2 years	Efficacy against infection: 100% (95% CI 65-100%)
Villa et al. 2005 (4)	Strains 16, 18, 6, and 11 (n=277) or placebo (n=275)	Young women	36 months	Combined incidence of infection with inoculated strains fell by 90% (95% CI 71-97%;P<0.001)
Harper et al. 2004 (5)	Strains 16 and 18 (n=1113)	Women aged 15-25 years	27 months	Efficacy of vaccine against: • incident infection was 91.6% (95% CI 64.5 to 98.0%) • persistent infection was 100% (95% CI 47 to 100%) • persistent cervical HPV infection was 95.1% • related cytological abnormalities was 92.9%

Please be aware that the above opinions are based upon review of abstracts of published articles and, therefore, no firm conclusions are offered. Because abstracts do not always accurately reflect the methods and findings of the full-length article or the limits on interpreting the published data, the reader is strongly encouraged to obtain the relevant articles before reaching conclusions about this technology. As such, ECRI has not evaluated the quality of these study designs, nor have we determined whether the authors used appropriate statistical methods to analyze their data. We are reluctant to comment on the reliability of these results in the absence of such evaluations. The purpose of this Hotline Response is to provide you with a summary of the literature based on our searches, and to give you information about what this technology is purported to accomplish. This Response is not intended to provide specific guidance for the care of individual patients.

Selected References

Note: In preparing the Hotline Response, information specialists research the topic and compile a <u>Bibliography</u>. We exclude individual case reports because they may not represent routine use. Technical articles are also excluded unless they include clinical trial results. In writing the Hotline Response analysts screen the <u>Bibliography</u> for references relevant to the topic, and these are provided below in the narrower list of <u>Selected References</u>.

References also include relevant ECRI content on your topic including ECRI documents that are not part of your HTAIS membership benefits. For an electronic copy of any non-HTAIS ECRI documents that are referenced in your Hotline Response, please contact the <u>Hotline Service</u>. For routine access to ECRI documents that are provided through other <u>ECRI Membership Services</u>, please contact <u>Don Cummins</u>.

1. ECRI. Concerns about human papillomavirus (HPV) vaccination [Hotline]. <u>ECRI</u>

2. Harper DM, Franco EL, Wheeler CM, Moscicki AB, Romanowski B, Roteli-Martins CM, Jenkins D, Schuind A, Costa Clemens SA, Dubin G. Sustained efficacy up to 4.5 years of a bivalent Ll virus-like particle vaccine against human papillomavirus types 16 and 18: follow-up from a randomised control trial. Lancet. 2006;367(95 18): 1247-55. <u>PubMed</u> 16631880 [PMID]

3. Mao C, Koutsky LA, Ault KA, Wheeler CM, Brown DR, Wiley DJ, Alvarez FB, Bautista OM, Jansen KU, Barr E. Efficacy of human papillomavirus—16 vaccine to prevent cervical intraepithelial neoplasia: a randomized controlled trial. Obstet Gynecol. 2006;l07(l):l8-27. <u>PubMed</u> 16394035 [PMID]

4. Villa LL, Costa RL, Petta CA, Andrade RP, Ault KA, Giuliano AR, Wheeler CM, Koutsky LA, Malm C, Lehtinen M, Skjeldestad FE, Olsson SE, Steinwall M, Brown DR, Kurman RJ, Roimett BM, Stoler MH, Ferenczy A, Harper DM, Tamms GM, Yu J, Lupinacci L, Railkar R, Taddeo FJ, Jansen KU, Esser MT, Sings HL, Saah AJ, Barr E. Prophylactic quadrivalent human papillomavirus (types 6, 11, 16, and 18) L1 virus-like particle vaccine in young women: a randomised double-blind placebo-controlled

multicentre phase II efficacy trial. Lancet Oncol. 2005;6(5):271-8. PubMed 15863374 [PMID]

5. Harper DM, Franco EL, Wheeler C, Ferris DG, Jenkins D, Schuind A, Zahaf T, Innis B, Naud P, De Carvalho NS, Roteli-Martins CM, Teixeira J, Blatter MM, Korn AP, Quint W, Dubin G. Efficacy of a bivalent L1 virus-like particle vaccine in prevention of infection with human papillomavims types 16 and 18 in young women: a randomised controlled trial. Lancet. 2004;364(9447):1757-65. PubMed 15541448 [PMID]

6. Pinto LA, Castle PE, Roden RB, Harro CD, Lowy DR, Schiller JT, Wallace D, Williams M, Kopp W, Frazer IH, Berzofsky JA, Hildesheim A. HPV-16 L1 VLP vaccine elicits a broad-spectrum of cytokine responses in whole blood. Vaccine. 2005;23(27):3555-64. PubMed 15855014 [PMID]

7. Poland GA, Jacobson RM, Koutsky LA, Tamms GM, Railkar R, Smith JF, Bryan JT, Cavanaugh PF Jr, Jansen KU, Barr E. Immunogenicity and reactogenicity of a novel vaccine for human papillomavirus 16: a 2-year randomized controlled clinical trial. Mayo Clin Proc. 2005;80(5):601-10. PubMed 15887427 [PMID]

8. Smith KL, Tristram A, Gallagher KM, Fiander AN, Man S. Epitope specificity and longevity of a vaccine-induced human T-cell response against HPV18. Int Immunol. 2005;17(2):167-76. PubMed 15623547 [PMID]

9. Ault KA, Giuliano AR, Edwards RP, Tamms G, Kim LL, Smith JF, Jansen KU, Allende M, Taddeo FJ, Skulsky D, Barr E. A phase I study to evaluate a human papillomavirus (HPV) type 18 Ll VLP vaccine. Vaccine. 2004;22(23-24):3004-7. PubMed 15297048 [PMID]

10. Fife KR, Wheeler CM, Koutsky LA, Barr E, Brown DR, Schiff MA, Kiviat NB, Jansen KU, Barber H, Smith JF, Tadesse A, Giacoletti K, Smith PR, Suhr G, Johnson DA. Dose-ranging studies of the safety and immunogenicity of human papillomavirus Type 11 and Type 16 virus-like particle candidate vaccines in young healthy women. Vaccine. 2004;22(2l-22):2943-52. PubMed 15246631

11. Pinto LA, Edwards J, Castle PE, Hano CD, Lowy DR, Schiller JT, Wallace D, Kopp W, Adelsberger JW, Baseler MW, Berzofsky JA, Hildesheim A. Cellular immune responses to human papillomavirus (HPV)-16 L1 in healthy volunteers immunized with recombinant HPV-16 L1 virus-like particles. J Infect Dis. 2003;188(2):327-38. PubMed 12854090 [PMID]

12. de Jong A, O'Neill T, Khan AY, Kwappenberg KM, Chisholm SE, Whittle NR, Dobson JA, Jack LC, St Clair Roberts JA, Offringa R, van der Burg SH, Hickling JK. Enhancement of human papillomavirus (HPV) type 16 E6 and E7-specific T-cell immunity in healthy volunteers through vac-

cination with TA-CIIN, an HPV16 L2E7E6 fusion protein vaccine. Vaccine. 2002;20(29-30):3456-64. PubMed 12297390 [PMID]

13. Emeny RT, Wheeler CM, Jansen KU, Hunt WC, Fu TM, Smith JF, MacMullen S, Esser MT, Paliard X. Priming of human papillomavirus type 11-specific humoral and cellular immune responses in college-aged women with a virus-like particle vaccine. J Virol. 2002;76(15):7832-42. PubMed 12097595 [PMID] Full text

14. Evans TG, Bonnez W, Rose RC, Koenig S, Demeter L, Suzich JA, O'Brien D, Campbell M, White WI, Baisley J, Reichman RC. A Phase 1 study of a recombinant virus like particle vaccine against human papillomavirus type 11 in healthy adult volunteers. J Infect Dis. 2001; 183(10): 1485-93. PubMed 11319684 [PMID]

15. Harro CD, Pang YY, Roden RB, Hildesheim A, Wang Z, Reynolds MJ, Mast TC, Robinson R, Murphy BR, Karron RA, Dillner J, Schiller JT, Lowy DR. Safety and immunogenicity trial in adult volunteers of a human papillomavirus 16 Ll virus-like particle vaccine. J Natl Cancer Inst. 2001;93(4):284-92. PubMed 11181775 [PMID] Full text

16. Giles M, Garland S. Human papillomavirus infection: An old disease, a new vaccine. Aust N Z J Obstet Gynaecol. 2006;46(3):180-5. PubMed 16704468 [PMID]

17. Stanley MA. Human papillomavirus vaccines. Rev Med Virol. 2006; 16(3):139-49. PubMed 16710836 [PMID]

18. Lowy DR, Schiller JT. Prophylactic human papillomavirus vaccines. J Clin Invest. 2006; 116(5): 1167-73. PubMed 16670757 [PMID] Full text

19. Crosbie EJ, Kitchener HC. Human papillomavirus in cervical screening and vaccination. Clin Sci (Lond). 2006; 11 0(5):543-52. PubMed 16597323 [PMID]

20. Monsonego J. [Cervical cancer prevention: the impact of HPV vaccination]. Gynecol Obstet Fertil. 2006;34(3): 189-201. PubMed 16529969 [PMIDJ

21. Feeley C. Advances in cervical cancer screening and human papillomavirus vaccines. J Br Menpause Soc. 2006;12(l):19-23. PubMed 16513018 [PMID]

22. Kahn JA. Vaccination as a prevention strategy for human papillomavims-related diseases. J Adolesc Health. 2005;37 (6 Suppl):S10-6. PubMed 16310136 [PMID]

23. Foerster V, Murtagh J. Vaccines for prevention of human papillo-

mavirus infection. Issues Emerg Health Technol. 2005;75:1-4. Pubmed 16544439 [PMID]

24. Campbell K. Preventing cervical cancer by vaccinating against HPV. Nurs Times. 2005;10l(46):21-2. PubMed 16315796 [PMID]

25. Govan VA. Strategies for human papillomavims therapeutic vaccines and other therapies based on the e6 and e7 oncogenes. Ann NY Acad Sci. 2005;1056:328-43. PubMed 16387699 [PMID]

26. Kahn JA, Bernstein DI. Human papillomavirus vaccines and adolescents. Curr Opin Obstet Gynecol. 2005; 1 7(5):476-82. PubMed 16141761 [PMID]

27. Villa LL. Prophylactic HPV vaccines: Reducing the burden of HPV-related diseases. Vaccine. 2005. PubMed 16194583 [PMID]

28. Simon P, Monnier S, Buxant F, Noel JC. [Anti-HPV vaccination against cervical cancer]. Rev Med Brux. 2005;26(5):433-8. PubMed 16318096 [PMID]

29. Scheurer ME, Tortolero-Luna G, Adler-Storthz K. Human papillomavirus infection: biology, epidemiology, and prevention. Int J Gynecol Cancer. 2005;15(5):727-46. PubMed 16174218 [PMID]

30. Sundar SS, Gornall RJ, Kehoe ST. Advances in the management of cervical cancer. J Br Menopause Soc. 2005;11(3):91-5. PubMed 16156999 [PMID]

31. Kadish AS, Einstein MH. Vaccine strategies for human papillomavirus-associated cancers. Cur Opin Oncol. 2005;17 (5):456-61. PubMed 16093795 [PMID]

32. Elbasha EH, Galvani AP. Vaccination against multiple HPV types. Math Biosci. 2005;197(1):88-117. PubMed 16095627 [PMID]

33. Denny L. The prevention of cervical cancer in developing countries. BJOG. 2005; 112(9): 1204-12. PubMed 16101597 [PMID]

34. Williamson AL, Passmore JA, Rybicki EP. Strategies for the prevention of cervical cancer by human papillomavirus vaccination. Best Pract Res Clin Obstet Gynaecol. 2005;19(4):531-44. PubMed 16150392 [PMID]

35. Mahdavi A, Monk BJ. Vaccines against human papillomavirus and cervical cancer: promises and challenges. Oncologist. 2005;10(7):528-38. PubMed 16079320 [PMID] Full text

36. Shew ML, Fortenberry JD. HPV infection in adolescents: natural history, complications, and indicators for viral typing. Semin Pediatr Infect Dis. 2005;16(3):168-74. PubMed 16044390 [PMID]

37. Hantz S, Alain S, Denis F. [Anti-papillomavirus vaccines and prevention of cervical cancer: progress and prospects]. Presse Med. 2005;34(10):745-53. PubMed 16026130 [PMID]

38. Leung AK, Kellner JD, Davies HD. Genital infection with human papillomavirus in adolescents. Adv Ther. 2005;22(3):187-97. PubMed 16236680 [PMID]

39. Bourgault-Villada I. [Vaccination against human papillomaviruses]. Therapie. 2005;60(3):27 1-4. PubMed 16128270 [PMID]

40. Franco EL, Harper DM. Vaccination against human papillomavirus infection: a new paradigm in cervical cancer control. Vaccine. 2005;23(17-18):2388-94. PubMed 15755633 [PMID]

41. Stem PL. Immune control of human papillomavims (HPV) associated anogenital disease and potential for vaccination. J Clin Virol. 2005; 32(Suppl l):S72-81. PubMed 15753015 [PMID]

42. Gravitt PE, Shah KV. A Virus-based Vaccine May Prevent Cervical Cancer. Curr Infect Dis Rep. 2005;7(2):l25-l3l. PubMed 15727740 [PMID]

43. Simon P. Progress towards a vaccine for cervical cancer. Curr Opin Obstet Gynecol. 2005;17(1):65-70 PubMed 15711414 [PMID]

44. Maclean J, Rybicki EP, Williamson AL. Vaccination strategies for the prevention of cervical cancer. Expert Rev Anticancer Ther. 2005;5(1):97-107. PubMed 15757442 [PMID]

45. Christensen ND. Emerging human papillomavirns vaccines. Expert Opin Emerg Drugs. 2005;10(1):5-19. PubMed 15757400 [PMID]

46. Valdespino-Gomez VM. [Preventive vaccines and immunotherapy clinical trials against cervical cancer]. Cir Cir. 2005;73(1): 57-69. PubMed 15888272 [PMID]

47. Santin AD, Bellone S, Roman JJ, Burnett A, Cannon MJ, Pecorelli S. Therapeutic vaccines for cervical cancer: dendritic cell-based immunotherapy. CurrPharm Des. 2005;11(27):3485-500. PubMed 16248803 [PMID]

48. Brinkman JA, Caffrey AS, Muderspach LI, Roman LD, Kast WM. The impact of anti HPV vaccination cervical cancer incidence and HPV induced cervical lesions: consequences for clinical management. Eur J Gynaecol Oncol. 2005;26(2):129-42. PubMed 15857016 [PMID]

49. Kang M, Lagakos SW. Evaluation of log-rank tests for infrequent observations from a multi-state process, with application to HPV vaccine efficacy. Stat Med. 2004;23(23):3681-96. PubMed 15534891 [PMID]

50. Joura EA. [Human papillomavirus and cervical cancer: presence and future of vaccination]. Gynalcol Geburtshilfliche Rundsch. 2004;44(3):142-5. PubMed 15211060 [PMID]

51. Franceschi S. [Human papillomavirus: a vaccine against cervical carcinoma uterine]. Epidemiol Prey. 2002;26(3): 140-4. PubMed 12197051 [PMID]

52. Gissmann L. [Possibilities of vaccination against HPV infections in cervix carcinoma]. Zentralbl Gynakol. 2001; 123(5):299-301. PubMed 11449623 [PMID]

53. Goldie SJ, Kohli M, Grima D, Weinstein MC, Wright TC, Bosch FX, Franco E. Projected clinical benefits and cost-effectiveness of a human papillomavirus 16/18 vaccine. J Natl Cancer Inst. 2004;96 (8):604-15. PubMed 15100338 [PMID] Full text

54. Kulasingam SL, Myers ER. Potential health and economic impact of adding a human papillomavirus vaccine to screening programs. JAMA. 2003;290(6):781-9. PubMed 12915431 [PMID]

55. Sanders GD, Taira AV. Cost-effectiveness of a potential vaccine for human papillomavirus. Emerg Infect Dis. 2003;90):37-48. PubMed 12533280 [PMID]

Search Summary:

The following databases were used to identify the literature and related materials. Please note that underlined titles are hyperlinked to the actual documents. For all search results, click on the title to access the document.

1. PubMed (National Library of Medicine) (www.pubmed.gov) (2001 through May 25, 2006)

Search Strategy:
S1 papillomavirus, human[mh] OR papillomavirus infections[mh]
S2 immunization[mh] OR vaccines[mh]
S3 "papilloma virus"[ti] OR "papilloma viruses"[ti] OR
    papillomavirus*[ti] OR hpv[ti] OR cervical[ti] OR cervix[ti]
S4 vaccin*[ti]
S5 (S1 AND S2) OR (S3 AND S4)

Results: There were 106 records identified. *These records are included in the Bibliography.*

2. The Cochrane Library (Published by John Wiley & Sons, Ltd.) (http://www.mrw.interscience.wiley.com/cochrane/) (2006, Issue 2) (2001 through May 25, 2006)

Search Strategy:
S1 "papilloma virus' OR "papilloma viruses" OR papillomavirus* OR hpv OR cervical OR cervix [in Record Title]
S2 vaccin* [in Record Title]
S3 S1 AND S2

Results: There were no unique bibliographic records; however the following full text document was identified. *(This document is also included in the Selected References list).*

- Canadian Coordinating Office for Health Technology Assessment (now Canadian Agency for Drugs and Technologies in Health CADTH). Foerster V, Murtagh J. Vaccines for prevention of human papillomavirus infection. *[Issues in Emerging Health Technologies Issue 75:2005].*

3. International Health Technology Assessment (1HTA) database (ECRI) (http://www.ta.ecri.org/IHTA/) (2001 through May 25, 2006)

Search Strategy:
(HPV OR "papilloma*") AND "vaccin*"; HPV AND (cervical OR cervix)

Results: There were no relevant records identified.

4. National Guideline Clearinghouse (NGC) Web site (www.guideline.gov) (2001 through May 25, 2006)

Search Strategy:
(HPV AND "papilloma*") AND vaccin*"; HPV

The following databases were used to identify the literature and related materials. Please note that underlined titles are hyperlinked to the actual documents. For all search results, click on the title to access the document.

Results: There were no documents mentioning HPV vaccines; however, there were numerous documents on other issues concerning HPV and cervical cancer. To access, search the NGC Web site using the search terms: *HPV*.

5. Healthcare Standards (HCS) database (ECRI)
(http://www.ta.ecri.org/hesf) (2001 through May 25, 2006)

Search Strategy:
(papillomavirus OR "sexually transmitted diseases") AND "vaccine*"; papillomavirus; "cervix neoplasms" OR "cervical intraepithelial neoplasms"

Results: There were no documents mentioning HPV vaccines; however, there were numerous documents on other issues concerning HPV and cervical cancer. To access, search the HCS database using the search terms: *HPV OR "cervix neoplasms"*.

6. U.S. Food and Drug Administration (FDA) Web site (www.fda.gov)
(June 12, 2006)

Search Strategy:
HPV AND vaccine; gardasil

Results: There following documents were identified.

• Center for Biologics Evaluation and Research (CBER). GARDASIL Product approval information - licensing action). [06/08/2006]. *(Note: includes links to Approval letter, Product label, and additional related documents).*

• Merck Research Laboratories. GARDASIL human papiliomavirus (types 6, 11, 1 6. 18) recombinant vaccine STN 125126. Briefing document. [04/18/2006, presented and approval recommended 05/18/2006].

• FDA statistical review and evaluation. Document for the Vaccines and Related Biological Products Advisory Committee (VRBPAC). [05/18/2006].

• VRBPAC background document. Gardasil HPV guadrivalent vaccine. [05/18/2006].

7. Centers for Medicare and Medicaid Services (CMS) Medicare Coverage Database (www.cms.hhs.gov/mcd/search.asp) (May 25, 2006)

Search Strategy:
HPV AND vaccine

Results: There were no national pending analyses or determinations identified; however, there were several local coverage policies which listed HPV vaccines under non-covered immunizations. To access, search the Local Coverage Database at: Medical Coverage Database *(Click Local Coverage, then select All States under Geographic area, then click Keyword, type:*

HPV immunization, click Entire Document, then click All Words (and) from the pull-down menu, and click Search).

8.   Selected Web Resources (June 12, 2006)

• Merck & Co., Inc. Gardasil [quadrivalent human papillomavirus (types 6, 11, 16, 18) recombinant vaccine]. [Cited 06/12/2006]. *(Note: includes links to patient information, prescribing information and additional related documents).*

• Centers for Disease Control and Prevention (CDC). HPV vaccine - CDC fact sheet. [Reviewed 04/2006]. *CDC National Immunization Program, Record of the meeting of the Advisory Committee on Immunization Practices.* [02/21-02/22/2006].

• American Social Health Association (ASHA). Gilbert L. Frequently asked questions about cervical cancer/HPV vaccine access in the U.S. *[05/2006].*

• National Cervical Cancer Coalition. Human papillomavirus (HPV). A status report on human papillomavirus vaccines. [Last modified 10/12/2005].

• Medscape. Mayeaux EJ, Spitzer M. Preventing cervical cancer and other HPV-related diseases. [Released 07/29/2005].

• National Cancer Institute (NCI). Human papiliomavirus and cancer: questions and answers. [Updated 05/17/2005]. Recent studies regarding FIPV and cervical cancer: questions and answers. [Posted 07/27/2005].

• ClinicalTrials.gov. [Cited 06/12/2006]. *(Note: there are numerous trials on HPV vaccines; to view, click link and enter the search terms: HPV, vaccine).*

Updated 06/13/2006

+Hayes search & summary

January 15, 2007

Platelet-Rich Plasma for Bone Healing and Fusion[2]

Search Strategy

A literature search of MEDLINE and EMBASE was completed on January 15, 2007, using the terms *platelet concentrate, platelet-rich plasma* combined with *spinal, fusion, bone AND fusion, bone healing, orthopedic surgery; platelet concentrate, platelet gel* combined with *orthopedic surgery, bone healing, spinal fusion.* The search was limited to English-language human clinical trials and review articles published in the last 5 years.

Description of Search Results

There is a small body of published literature available related to platelet-rich plasma (PRP) for bone healing and fusion. Twelve abstracts were found, including 1 randomized controlled trial (n=10), 7 clinical studies (n=20 to 180), and 1 case report (n=3). In addition, 2 review articles and 1 article comparing different commercially available methods of point-of-care platelet gel preparation were also retrieved. The clinical studies described the use of PRP for various orthopedic procedures, including tibial osteotomy, foot and ankle surgery, total ankle arthroplasty, Charcot's foot reconstruction, total knee arthroplasty, and lumbar fusion.

Regulatory Agency Information

Administration of PRP is a procedure and is, therefore, not subject to regulation by the Food and Drug Administration (FDA). However, the devices used to prepare PRP are regulated by the FDA premarket approval process. Several centrifuge devices have been approved by the FDA for preparation of PRP. The GPS® Platelet Separation Kit (Biomet Inc.) is one example of an approved centrifuge device associated in the literature with the use of PRP for orthopedic applications.

Biomet Inc. received 510(k) approval (K030555) for the GPS Platelet Separation Kit on April 11, 2003. It is designed for use in the clinical laboratory or intraoperatively at the point of care, for the safe and effective preparation of platelet-poor plasma and platelet concentrate from a small sample (50-60 ml) of whole blood.

Below are some of the centrifuge devices approved for platelet separation listed in the FDA 510(k) database. A full list of approved centrifuge devices can be found at the FDA site by inserting **JQC** into the **Product code** field of the form found at this link: http://www.accessdata.fda.gov/scripts/cdrh/cf-docs/cfPMN/pmn.cfm.

FDA Approvals
   Enter **510(k) number** at this site: http://www.accessdata.fda.gov/scripts/cdrh/cfdocs/cfPMN/pmn.cfm.

---

[2]Reprinted, with permission, from *Winifed S. Hayes, Inc.* 2007. Copyright 2007 by Winifred S. Hayes, Inc.

K030555: GPS Platelet Separation Kit (Biomet Inc.) approved on April 11, 2003
K021902: Magellan® Autologous Platelet Separator (Medtronic Inc.) approved on August 12, 2002
K991430: SmartPReP® Centrifuge System (Harvest Technologies LLC) approved on May 28, 1999

No Centers for Medicare & Medicaid Services (CMS) National Coverage Determination was found for PRP for bone healing and fusion.

Conclusions

There is sufficient evidence to assess the safety and efficacy of PRP for bone healing for ankle indications. An assessment of this technology will be provided in a Hayes Health Technology Brief and/or Hayes Medical Technology Directory report as permitted by our production schedule, with priority given to frequently requested topics.

Other Relevant Information

Of the estimated 5.6 million fractures that occur annually in the United States, approximately 5% to 10% will demonstrate signs of impaired healing, which results in either delayed union or nonunion of the fracture. PRP contains growth factors that maybe useful in healing nonunion fractures. Also known as platelet gel, or platelet concentrate, PRP is a blood product that is created by isolating and concentrating platelets from the patient's own blood. A centrifuge is used in this process to separate the blood into layers; the middle layer, or "buffy coat," contains plasma with concentrated platelets.

PRP contains many growth factors, including platelet-derived growth factor (PDGF), transforming growth factor (TGF-beta1), insulin-like growth factor-1 (IGF-I), and vascular endothelial growth factor (VEGF). These proteins may promote bone formation, but they are not universally recognized to be osteoinductive, or capable of inducing new bone growth. PRP may be mixed with bone grafting materials or applied during orthopedic surgery, with the hope it will facilitate the bone healing process. Currently, PRP is generally used as a graft extender and not as a replacement for the actual bone graft.

Manufacturer Sites:
Listed below are some manufacturers of centrifuge devices. NOTE: Harvest Technologies Corp. is the manufacturer of the SmartPReP Centrifuge System, which is the antecedent device to the Symphony II Platelet Concentrate System. DePuy Spine purchased the marketing and distribution rights for the Symphony II device in 2000.
Biomet Inc.: http://www.biomet.com/
Gravitational Platelet Separation (GPS) System info: http://www.bmetbiologics.com/index.cfm
Information download for GPS System: http://www.biometbiologics.com/downloads.cfm

DePuy Spine (a Johnson & Johnson company): http://www.depuyspine.
com/home.asp
  Symphony II Platelet Concentrate System info: http://www.depuyspine.
  com/products/biologicssolutions/ii.asp
  Symphony II Platelet Concentrate System product insert: http://www.
  depuyspine.com/ds_products_syndication/packageinserts/0902_90_
  022.pdf
Harvest Technologies LLC: http://www.harvesttech.com/index.htm
  SmartPReP Platelet Concentrate System: http://www.harvesttech.com/
  IntlPRP_OLD.htm
Medtronic Inc.: http://www.medtronic.com/
  Magellan Autologous Platelet Separator: http://www.medtronic.com/
  cardsurgery/bloodmgmt/magellan_ovrw.html

Payer Coverage Policies:
  Three payer coverage policies were located that refer to the use of PRP in
  bone healing. All policies consider its use experimental and investigational
  or unproven for bone healing and other orthopedic indications.
  Aetna: http://www.aetna.com/cpb/medical/datal400_ 499/0411.html
  CIGNA HealthCare: http://www.cigna.com/health/provider/
  medical/procedural/coverage_positions/medical/mm_ 0068_
  coveragepositioncriteria_woundhealing.pdf
  Regence Group: http://www.regence.com/trgmedpol/medicine/med77.html

Online Articles:
  Percutaneous injection of autogenous growth factors in patient with
  nonunion of the humerus. A case report (Bielecki and Gazdzik, 2006),
  Journal of Orthopaedics: http:llwww.jortho.org1200613131e15/index.htm
  Treatment of recalcitrant enthesopathy of the hip with platelet rich plasma
  — a report of three cases (Scioli M, 2006), Clinical Orthopaedic Society
  News (NOTE: Article is on pages 6-7): http://www.bmetbiologics.corn/
  international/print/Scioli_newsletter_submission.pdf
  Overview of bone grafting (2002), Medscape Today: http://www.medscape.
  com/viewarticle/4439021

  A comprehensive search of the Internet did not return any information regarding evidence-based practice guidelines or ongoing clinical trials for PRP for
  bone healing and fusion.

Search Results with Abstracts
January 15, 2007
MEDLINE, EMBASE
Search terms: *platelet concentrate, platelet-rich plasma combined with spinal,
fusion, bone AND fusion, bone healing, orthopedic surgery,
platelet concentrate, platelet gel combined with orthopedic surgery, bone healing, spinal fusion*
Search limits: English-language human clinical trials and review articles published in the last 5 years

Search yield: 14 citations
Retrieved: 12 abstracts

1: Foot & Ankle International. 27(12):1079-85, 2006 Dec.

Arthroscopic ankle arthrodesis: factors influencing union in 39 consecutive patients.

Collman DR. Kaas MH. Schuberth JM.

Department of Orthopaedic Surgery, Kaiser Permanente Medical Group, Modesto, CA, USA.

BACKGROUND: Arthroscopic ankle arthrodesis is an effective alternative to open techniques with established advantages in select patient populations. The purpose of this study was to evaluate patients who had arthroscopic ankle arthrodesis for end-stage arthritis with minimal to no deformity of the ankle and to report factors influencing union. METHODS: Thirty-nine consecutive patients had arthroscopic ankle arthrodesis between 1994 and 2003. Clinical records and radiographs were retrospectively reviewed to evaluate variable that could predispose patients to nonunion. Union outcomes were correlated with etiology of arthritis, ankle deformity, medical co-morbidities, and the use of demineralized bone matrix or platelet-rich plasma. Arthroscopic ankle arthrodesis was accomplished with a consistent technique using crossed transmalleolar cannulated screw fixation. RESULTS: Thirty-four of 39 patients (87.2%) achieved radiographic and clinical union. The average time to fusion was 47 (range 37 to 70) days. Poor bone quality and inherent positional ankle deformity were identified as risk factors for nonunion. Patients who smoked, had diabetes rnellitus, peripheral neuropathy, or other medical co-morbidities attained ankle union in nearly all cases, In obese patients, there was an observed trend towards ankle nonunion (relative risk 5.81, p = 0.049, Fishers Exact test). The addition of demineralized bone matrix or platelet-rich plasma did not improve the rate of ankle union. Aside from nonunion, 10 patients developed minor complications. CONCLUSION: Arthroscopic ankle arthrodesis achieves high union rates, facilitates short time to union, and permits rapid patient mobility. Careful patient selection is important for the procedure. Synthetic allograft or platelet-rich plasma did not enhance the fusion rate. Obese patients showed a trend towards nonunion in this series.

UI: 17207436

2: Journal of Extra-Corporeal Technology. 38(2):174-87. 2005 Jun.

Platelet-rich plasma and platelet gel: a review.

Everts PA. Knape JT. Weibrich C. Schonberger JR. Hoffmann J. Overdevest EP. Box HA. van Zundert A.

Department of Extra Corporeal Blood Management, Catharina Hospital, Eindhoven, The Netherlands. everts@elive.nl

Strategies to reduce blood loss and transfusion of allogeneic blood products during surgical procedures are important in modern times. The most important and well-known autologous techniques are preoperative autologous predonation, hemodilution, perioperative red cell salvage, postoperative wound blood autotransfusion, and pharmacologic modulation of the hemostatic process. At present, new developments in the preparation of preoperative autologous blood component therapy by whole blood platelet-rich plasma (PRP) and platelet-poor plasma (PPP) sequestration have evolved, This technique has been proven to reduce the number of allogeneic blood transfusions during open heart surgery and orthopedic operations. Moreover, platelet gel and fibrin sealant derived from PRP and PPP mixed with thrombin, respectively, can be exogenously applied to tissues to promote wound healing, bone growth, and tissue sealing. However, to our disappointment, not many well-designed scientific studies are available, and many anecdotic stories exist, whereas questions remain to be answered. We therefore decided to study perioperative blood management in more detail with emphasis on the application and production of autologous platelet gel and the use of fibrin sealant. This review addresses a large variety of aspects relevant to platelets, platelet-rich plasma, and the application of platelet gel. In addition, an overview of recent animal and human studies is presented.

Publication Types:
  Review
UI: 16921694

3:   Advances in Therapy. 23(2):218-37, 2006 Mar-Apr.

Autologous platelet-rich plasma for wound and osseous healing: a review of the literature and commercially available products.

Roukis TS. Zgonis T. Tiernan B.

Limb Preservation Service, Department of Vascular Surgery MCHJ-SV, Madigan Army Medical Center, Tacoma, Washington 98431, USA.

The application of autologous platelets that have been sequestered, concentrated, and mixed with thrombin to create growth factor-concentrated, autologous platelet-rich plasma for application to soft tissue wounds and for osseous healing has been a subject of great interest for much of the past 2 decades. Autologous platelet-rich plasma, which consists of both quantitative and qualitative components, has the greatest potency or ability to produce the desired effect. Manufacturers prepare autologous platelet-rich plasma with the ultimate goal of maximizing its benefits while minimizing potential risks, Unfortunately, the manufacturing processes for autologous platelet-rich plasma are highly variable, and the types of proprietary systems available on the market for soft tissue and osseous applications are numerous. The authors provide here an in-depth review of commercially available systems for delivery of autologous platelet-rich plasma that emphasizes the subtle yet important differences among systems. In addition, a detailed review of the literature regarding the use of autologous platelet-rich plasma in soft tissue and osseous healing is provided. Although findings are not yet conclusive, autologous platelet-rich plasma has been shown to be safe, reproducible, and effective in mimicking the natural processes of soft tissue wound and osseous healing.

Publication Types:
Research Support, Non-U.S. Gov't
Review
UI: 16751155

4: Journal of Biomedical Materials Research. Part B, Applied Biomaterials. 76(2):364-72, 2006 Feb.

Evaluation of bone healing enhancement by lyophilized bone grafts supplemented with platelet gel: a standardized methodology in patients with tibial osteotomy for genu varus.

Savarino L. Cenni F. Tarabusi C. Dallari D. Stagni C. Cenacchi A. Fornasari PM. Giunti A. Baldini N.

Laboratory for Pathophysiology of Orthopaedic Implants, Istituti Ortopedioi Rizzoli, Via di Barbiano 1/10, 40136 Bologna, Italy. lucia.savarino@ior.it

Orthopedic practice may be adversely affected by an inadequate bone repair that might compromise the success of surgery. In recent years, new approaches have been sought to improve bone healing by accelerating the rate of new bone formation and the maturation of the matrix. There is currently great interest in procedures involving the use of platelet gel (PG) to improve tissue healing, with satisfactory results both in vitro and in maxillofacial surgery. Otherwise, to our knowledge, only a preliminary clinical study was undertaken in the orthopedic field [Kitoh et al., Bone 2004;35:892-898] and the efficacy of PG is still controversial. Our paper focuses on the effect on bone regeneration by adding PG to lyophilized bone chips used for orthopedic applications. The clinical model and the laboratory methodology were standardized. As a clinical model, we employed the first series of patients of a randomized case-control study undergoing high tibial osteotomy (HTO) for genu varus. Ten subjects were enrolled: in 5 patients lyophilized bone chips supplemented with PG were inserted during tibial osteotomy (group A); 5 patients were used as a control (group B) and lyophilized bone chips without gel were applied. Forty-five days after surgery, computed tomography scan guided biopsies of grafted areas were obtained and the bone maturation was evaluated by a standardized methodology: the Osteogenic and angiogenio processes were semi-quantitatively characterized by using histomorphometry, and the mineral component of the lyophilized and host bone was analyzed by using X-ray diffraction technique with sample microfocusing and miororadiography. Lyophilized bone with PG seems to accelerate the healing process, as shown by new vessel formation and deposition of newly formed bone, with no evidence of inflammatory cell infiltrate, when compared with lyophilized bone without gel. On the contrary, lyophilized bone undergo a resorption process, and a fibrous tissue often fills the spaces between chips. A histio-cytic/giant-cell reaction is sometimes present. Otherwise, no differences have been found concerning microstructure. Our findings show the reliability of the methodology used to monitor early bone repair. The completion of the study and the evaluation of the ultimate clinical outcome are necessary in order to verify PG in vivo effects in orthopedic surgery.

Publication Types:
    Randomized Controlled Trial
UI: 16161123

5: Journal of Surgical Orthopaedic Advances, 14(1):I7-22, 2005.

Union rates using autologous platelet concentrate alone and with bone graft in high-risk foot and ankle surgery patients.

Bibbo C. Bono CM. Lin SS.

Department of Orthopaedic Surgery, Marshiceld Clinic, 1000 North Oak Avenue, Marshfield, WI 54449, USA. bibbo.christopher@marshfieldclinic.org

Adjuvant use of autologous platelet concentrate (APC) to assist bone healing in foot and ankle surgery has not been reported. This study examined the clinical results and complications after the adjuvant use of APC in high-risk patients undergoing elective foot and ankle surgery. Patients at risk for bone-healing complications were prospectively enrolled over a 6-month period for the intraoperative application of APC. Patients were followed every 2 weeks for radiographic union and complications. Sixty-two high-risk patients were enrolled, totaling 123 procedures. Mean patient age was 51 years (range, 16-76), there were 36 females and 26 males, and 24 patients were smokers. Overall, a 94% union rate was achieved at a mean of 41 days. For APC alone, the mean time to union was 40 days; when APC was used with autograft, the mean time to union was 45 days (p = .173, two-tailed t-test). These data suggest that adjuvant APC results in an acceptable time to union and may be a useful adjunct to promote osseous healing in high-risk patients undergoing elective foot and ankle surgery.

UI: 15766437

6: Foot Ankle Int. 2005 Oct;26(I0):640-6.

The use of autologous concentrated growth factors to promote syndesmosis fusion in the Agility total ankle replacement. A preliminary study.

Coetzee JC, Pomeroy GC, Watts JD, Barrow C.

Department of Orthopaedic Surgery, University of Minnesota R200, 2450 Riverside Avenue South, Minneapolis, MN 55454, USA. Coetz001@tc.umn.edu

BACKGROUND: The Agility (DePuy, Warsaw, Indiana) total ankle replacement has been in use since 1984. One of the most common complications continues to be delayed union or nonunions of the distal tibiofibular syndesmosis. In the 1999, 114 Agility total ankle replacements were done at two centers in the United States without the use of autologous reported studies on the Agility ankle the delayed union and nonunion rate can be as high as 38%. METHODS: Since concentrated growth factors. Since July of 2001, 66 Agility ankles were implanted with Symphony (DePuy, Warsaw, Indiana) augmented bone grafting. The standard operative technique was followed in all the patients. Prospective data was collected on all patients. The standard ankle radiographs were taken preoperatively and postoperative at 8 weeks, 12 weeks, 16 weeks, 6 months, and yearly. CT scans were obtained at 6 months if fusion at the syndesmosis was questionable, The Graphpad Instat software (Graphpad Software Inc., San Diego, CA) was used for statistical analysis. The two-tailed unpaired t-test was used, and the value <0.05 was considered significant. RESULTS: There was no statistical difference in the demographic data for the two groups. In 114 ankle replacements without autologous concentrated growth factors 70 fused at 8 weeks (61%), 14 fused at 12 weeks (12%), 13 fused at 6 months (12%). There were 17 nonunions (15%); delayed unions (3 to 6 months) and nonunions, therefore, equaled 27%. The syndesmosis fused in 50 of the 66 ankle replacements (76%) that had autologous concentrated growth fractures at 8 weeks (76%); 12 fused at 3 months (18%). 2 fused at 6 months (3%), 2 had nonunions (3%). Delayed unions (3 to 6 months) and nonunions equaled 6%. There was a statistically significant improvement in the 8- and 12-week fusion rates, and a statistically significant reduction in delayed unions and nonunions. CONCLUSION: Autologous concentrated growth factors appear to make a significant positive difference in the syndesmosis union rate in total ankle replacements.

Publication Types:
    Comparative Study
PMID: 16221457 [PubMed - indexed for MEDLINE]

7:    Foot & Ankle International. 26(6):458-61, 2005 Jun.

Enhancement of syndesmotic fusion rates in total ankle arthroplasty with the use of autologous platelet concentrate,

Barrow CR. Pomeroy GC.

Orthopaedic Specialty of Spokane, 785 East Holland Avenue, Spokane, WA 99218, USA.
cbarrow@orthospecialtyclinic.com

BACKGROUND: One of the challenges of total ankle arthroplasty continues to be achieving a solid distal fusion of the tibiotibular joint. Delayed union rates of 29% to 38% and the nonunion rates of 9% to 18% for syndesmotic fusion have been documented. The risk of tibial component migration has been reported to increase 8.5 times if a solid syndesmotic fusion is absent. Growth factors have been shown to accelerate bone healing and may enhance the fusion of the syndesmosis and, thereby, decrease the frequency of nonunion and subsequent tibial component migration. METHODS: An autologous platelet concentrate was used to increase the amount of growth factors at the site of the distal tibiofibular joint fusion in 20 total ankle arthroplasties. RESULTS: Our 6-month fusion rate was 100%. When compared to historical controls (6-month fusion rate of 62%) the difference was statistically significant (p CONCLUSION: The improved rate of distal tibiofibular fusion may be attributable to the increased presence of growth factors provided by an autologous platelet concentrate.

UI: 15960912

8:   Spine. 30(9):E243-6; discussion E247. 2005 May 1.

Platelet gel (AGF) fails to increase fusion rates in instrumented posterolateral fusions.

Carreon LY. Glassman SD. Anekstein Y. Puno RM.

Leatherman Spine Center, Louisville, Kentucky 40202, USA.
lcarreon@spinemds.com

STUDY DESIGN: Retrospective cohort study. OBJECTIVE: To determine the effect on fusion of adding platelet gel to autologous iliac crest graft. SUMMARY OF BACKGROUND DATA: Platelet gel is an osteoinductive material prepared by ultra-concentration of platelets and contains multiple growth factors. Proprietary commercial methods are available for harvesting autologous platelet gel concentrates for use as graft supplement in spine fusions. METHODS: We reviewed 76 consecutive patients who underwent instrumented posterolateral lumbar fusion with autologous iliac crest bone graft mixed with autologous growth factor (AGF). A control group was randomly selected from patients who underwent instrumented posterolateral lumbar fusion with autologous bone graft alone. The groups were matched for age, sex, smoking history, and number of levels fused. Demographic, surgical, and clinical data were collected from medical records. Diagnosis of nonunion was based on exploration during revision surgery or evidence of nonunion on computerized tomography. The Fisher exact test was used to compare fusion rates. RESULTS: In both groups, mean age was 50 years, and 24% were smokers. The nonunion rate was 25% in the AGF group and 17% in the control group. This difference was not statistically significant (P= 0.18). CONCLUSIONS: Platelet gel preparation requires blood draws from the patient. This procedure adds to the risk and cost of surgery. The technique for AGF harvest evaluated in this study provides the highest concentration of platelets among the commercially available methods. Despite this, we showed that platelet gel failed to enhance fusion rate when added to autograft in patients undergoing instrumented posterolateral spinal fusion. The authors do not recommend the use of platelet gel to supplement autologous bone graft during instrumented posterolateral spinal fusion.

Publication Types:
    Research Support. Non-U.S. Gov't
UI: 15864142

9:   Clinics in Podiatric Medicine & Surgery. 22(4):561-84, vi, 2005 Oct.

The utilization of autologous growth factors for the facilitation of fusion in complex neuropathic fractures in the diabetic population.

Grant WP. Jerlin EA. Pietrzak WS. Tam HS.

Tidewater Foot and Ankle Center, 762 Independence Blvd., Suite 771, Virginia Beach, VA 23455, USA.
charcotking@yahoo.com

A review of current knowledge of autologous growth factors as used in foot and ankle surgery is presented. This knowledge is clinically correlated with 50 Charcot's foot reconstruction patients who had diabetes and who were randomized to a platelet-rich plasma (PRP) concentration system (Symphony, DePuy, Warsaw, Indiana) or a hollow-fiber hemoconcentration system (Interpore Cross AGF, Interpore Cross, Irvine, California) trial. Although the literature supports the notion that Symphony produces a higher yield of intact platelets mole consistently, clinically, a statistically significantly higher number of patients treated with Interpore Cross AGF went onto solid fusion. The findings may indicate that one type of PRP may be indicated for a particular clinical circumstance based on the patient's medical history and resultant local wound environment.

Publication Types:
    Case Reports
    Comparative Study
    Review
UI: 16213380

10: Bone. 35(4):892-8, 2004 Oct.

Transplantation of marrow-derived mesenchymal stem cells and platelet-rich plasma during distraction osteogenesis—a preliminary result of three cases.

Kitoh H. Kitakoji T. Tsuchiya H. Mitsuyama H. Nakamura H. Katoh M. Ishiguro N.

Department of Orthopaedic Surgery, Nagoya University School of Medicine, Showa-ku, Nagoya, Aichi 466-8550, Japan. hkitoh@med.nagoya-u.ac.jp

Clinical results of distraction osteogenesis with transplantation of marrow-derived mesenchymal stem cells (MSCs) and platelet-rich plasma (PRP) were reviewed in three femora and two tibiae of the two patients with achondroplasia and one patient with congenital pseudarthrosis of the tibia. MSCs derived from the iliac crest were cultured with osteogenic supplements and differentiated into osteoblast-like cells. PRP, which is known to contain several

growth factors and coagulate immediately by a minute introduction of thrombin and calcium, was prepared just before transplantation. Culture-expanded
osteoblast-like coils and autologous PRP were injected into the distracted
callus with the thrombin-calcium mixture so that the PRP gel might develop
within the injected site. Transplantation of MSCs and PRP was done at the
lengthening and consolidation period in each patient. The target lengths were
obtained in every leg without major complications and the average healing
index was 23.0 days/cm (18.8-26.9 days/cm). Although these results are still
preliminary, transplantation of osteoblast-like cells and PRP, which seemed
to be a safe and minimally invasive cell therapy, could shorten the treatment
period by acceleration of bone regeneration during distraction osteogenesis.

Publication Types:
    Case Reports
    Research Support, Non-U.S. Gov't
UI: 15454096

11: Journal of Spinal Disorders & Techniques. 1 7(5):380-4, 2004 Oct.

Role of activated growth factors in lumbar spinal fusions.

Castro EP Jr.

Tulane Health Sciences, New Orleans, Louisiana. fcastro@seortho.com

BACKGROUND: The concentration of platelets into an activated growth factor
(AGF) gel may stimulate graft consolidation into a fusion mass. Preoperative
hemodilution and intraoperative clot activation may also reduce the overall
blood loss. Consequently, the need for postoperative transfusions may also
be reduced. OBJECTIVE: The objective of this work was to report our experience with AGF platelet gels in transforaminal lumbar interbody fusion (TLIF)
procedures. METHODS: A consecutive series of patients between 1996 and
1999 undergoing one- and two-level TLIFs with AGF were compared with a
consecutive series of TLIF patients who did not receive AGF. Sixty-two control subjects who did not receive AGF and 22 patients who received an AGF
platelet gel were compared after 41 and 34 months of follow-up, respectively.
RESULTS: On average, the AGF group required 18 minutes of additional
preincision anesthesia (P = 0.0001). No statistical differences in the operative
times, estimated blood loss, postoperative drainage, percentage of patients
requiring a transfusion, or length of hospitalization were appreciated between
the two groups. The 19% decrease in the arthrodesis rate of the AGF group,
as compared with the control group, did not reach statistical significance.
Platelet counts from the AGF platelet concentrates demonstrated an average
3.5-fold increase compared with preoperative serum levels. CONCLUSIONS:
The theoretical benefits of AGF platelet gel technology were not clinically appreciated. The cost of implementing this technology may therefore outweigh
its theoretical benefits.

Publication Types:
  Clinical Trial
  Comparative Study
  Controlled Clinical Trial
UI: 15385877

12: Journal of Extra-Corporeal Technology. 36(I):28-35, 2004 Mar

Comparison of methods for point of care preparation of autologous platelet gel.

Kevy SV. Jacobson MS.

Harvard Medical School, Director Emeritus, Transfusion Service, Children's Hospital and CBR Laboratories, Boston, Massachusetts 02115, USA.

A platelet gel (PG) is produced by the addition of calcium chloride and thrombin to a platelet concentrate (PC). PG releases multiple growth factors, which have the ability to initiate and stimulate one growth factor's function in the presence of others. This finding has resulted in the use of PG in orthopedic, plastic, and reconstructive surgery. The study compared the commercial systems available for the preparation of PG. All procedures were performed according to the manufacturers directions. The devices were evaluated with respect to ease of use, collection efficiency, platelet quality, and growth factor release. The SmartPReP requires only four processing steps compared to 12 to 24 required by other devices. The SmartPReP and the CATS were the most reproducible, as evidenced by their low coefficient of variation of 13% and 16%. The mean platelet yield was 72% for the SmartPReP, 58% for the 3iPCCS, 54% for the Sequestra, 31% for the Secquire, 31% for the CATS, 27% for the Interpore Cross, and 42.6% for the Biomet OPS. The mean total amount of PDGF-AB and TGF-B1 obtained from the SmartPReP is greater than other systems evaluated. The SmartPReP produced a consistent PC with a yield that was four times baseline range with the lowest coefficient of variation.

Publication Types:
  Comparative Study
  Research Support, Non-U.S. Gov't
UI: 15095838

Appendix F

Guideline Standards:
The AGREE Instrument
and COGS Checklist

THE APPRAISAL OF GUIDELINES RESEARCH AND EVALUATION (AGREE) INSTRUMENT[1]

Scope and Purpose

1. The overall objective(s) of the guideline is (are) specifically described.
2. The clinical question(s) covered by the guideline is (are) specifically described.
3. The patients to whom the guideline is meant to apply are specifically described.

Stakeholder Involvement

4. The guideline development group includes individuals from all the relevant professional groups.
5. The patients' views and preferences have been sought.
6. The target users of the guideline are clearly defined.
7. The guideline has been piloted among target users.

Rigour of Development

8. Systematic methods were used to search for evidence.
9. The criteria for selecting the evidence are clearly described.
10. The methods used for formulating the recommendations are clearly described.

---

[1]Reprinted in adapted format, with permission, from the *AGREE Research Trust* http://www.agreetrust.org. Copyright 2006 by the AGREE Research Trust.

11. The health benefits, side effects and risks have been considered in formulating the recommendations.
12. There is an explicit link between the recommendations and the supporting evidence.
13. The guideline has been externally reviewed by experts prior to its publication.
14. A procedure for updating the guideline is provided.

Clarity and Presentation

15. The recommendations are specific and unambiguous.
16. The different options for management of the condition are clearly presented.
17. Key recommendations are easily identifiable.
18. The guideline is supported with tools for application.

Applicability

19. The potential organisational barriers in applying the recommendations have been discussed.
20. The potential cost implications of applying the recommendations have been considered.
21. The guideline presents key review criteria for monitoring and/or audit purposes.

Editorial Independence

22. The guideline is editorially independent from the funding body.
23. Conflicts of interest of guideline development members have been recorded.

CONFERENCE ON GUIDELINES STANDARDIZATION (COGS) CHECKLIST FOR REPORTING CLINICAL PRACTICE GUIDELINES[2]

Topic	Description
1. Overview material	Provide a structured abstract that includes the guideline's release date, status (original, revised, updated), and print and electronic sources.
2. Focus	Describe the primary disease/condition and intervention/service/technology that the guideline addresses. Indicate any alternative preventive, diagnostic or therapeutic interventions that were considered during development.
3. Goal	Describe the goal that following the guideline is expected to achieve, including the rationale for development of a guideline on this topic.
4. Users/setting	Describe the intended users of the guideline (e.g., provider types, patients) and the settings in which the guideline is intended to be used.
5. Target population	Describe the patient population eligible for guideline recommendations and list any exclusion criteria.
6. Developer	Identify the organization(s) responsible for guideline development and the names/credentials/potential conflicts of interest of individuals involved in the guideline's development.
7. Funding source/sponsor	Identify the funding source/sponsor and describe its role in developing and/or reporting the guideline. Disclose potential conflict of interest.
8. Evidence Collection	Describe the methods used to search the scientific literature, including the range of dates and databases searched, and criteria applied to filter the retrieved evidence.

[2]Reprinted, with permission, from *Annals of Internal Medicine* 2003. Copyright 2007 by the American College of Physicians.

Topic	Description
9. Recommendation grading criteria	Describe the criteria used to rate the quality of evidence that supports the recommendations and the system for describing the strength of the recommendations. Recommendation strength communicates the importance of adherence to a recommendation and is based on both the quality of the evidence and the magnitude of anticipated benefits or harms.
10. Method for synthesizing evidence	Describe how evidence was used to create recommendations, e.g., evidence tables, meta-analysis, decision analysis.
11. Prerelease review	Describe how the guideline developer reviewed and/or tested the guidelines prior to release.
12. Update plan	State whether or not there is a plan to update the guideline and, if applicable, an expiration date for this version of the guideline.
13. Definitions	Define unfamiliar terms and those critical to correct application of the guideline that might be subject to misinterpretation.
14. Recommendations and rationale	State the recommended action precisely and the specific circumstances under which to perform it. Justify each recommendation by describing the linkage between the recommendation and its supporting evidence. Indicate the quality of evidence and the recommendation strength, based on the criteria described in 9.
15. Potential benefits and harms	Describe anticipated benefits and potential risks associated with implementation of guideline recommendations.
16. Patient preferences	Describe the role of patient preferences when a recommendation involves a substantial element of personal choice or values.
17. Algorithm	Provide (when appropriate) a graphical description of the stages and decisions in clinical care described by the guideline.

Topic	Description
18. Implementation considerations	Describe anticipated barriers to application of the recommendations. Provide reference to any auxiliary documents for providers or patients that are intended to facilitate.

REFERENCES

The AGREE Collaboration. 2001. *The Appraisal of Guidelines for Research and Evaluation (AGREE) Instrument*. London, UK: The AGREE Research Trust http://www.agreetrust.org/docs/AGREE_Instrument_English.pdf (accessed September 2007).

Shiffman, R. N., P. Shekelle, M. Overhage, J. Slutsky, J. Grimshaw, and A. M. Deshpande. 2003. Standardized reporting of clinical practice guidelines: A proposal from the Conference on Guideline Standardization. *Annals of Internal Medicine* 139(6):493-500.

Appendix G

Committee Biographies

Barbara J. McNeil, M.D., Ph.D., *Chair*, is the Ridley Watts Professor and founding Head of the Department of Health Care Policy at Harvard Medical School. She is also a professor of radiology at Harvard Medical School and at Brigham and Women's Hospital. Dr. McNeil's research activities focus on several areas related to quality of care and technology assessment. For several years she coordinated large-scale studies comparing the value of alternative imaging modalities for several cancers. Her most recent projects involve comparing the quality of care for veterans with cancer to the quality of care provided to Medicare beneficiaries seen in private settings. She is currently working with the national Blue Cross and Blue Shield Association to evaluate the effectiveness of various interventions that its plans have undertaken to increase quality and decrease cost. Dr. McNeil received an A.B. from Emmanuel College, an M.D. from Harvard Medical School, and a Ph.D. from Harvard University. She is a member of the Institute of Medicine of the National Academies and the American Academy of Arts and Sciences. Dr. McNeil is also a member of the Blue Cross Technology Evaluation Commission; the Medicare Evidence Development Coverage Advisory Committee, of which she is chair; and the Council for Performance Measurement for the Joint Commission. Previously, Dr. McNeil served as a member of the Prospective Payment Assessment Commission and the Publications Committee of the *New England Journal of Medicine*.

Harold C. Sox, M.D., M.A.C.P., *Vice Chair*, editor of the *Annals of Internal Medicine*, received an undergraduate degree from Stanford University in 1961 and a medical degree from Harvard Medical School in 1966. After serving as a medical intern and resident at Massachusetts General Hospital, he spent two years doing research at the National Institutes of Health and three years at Dartmouth Medical School where he began his studies of medical decision making. Dr. Sox then spent 15 years at the Stanford University School of Medicine as chief of the Division of General Internal Medicine and as a director of ambulatory care at the Palo Alto Veterans Administration Medical Center. In 1988, he returned to Dartmouth Medical School to chair the Department of Medicine as the Joseph M. Huber Professor of Medicine until 2001, when he became editor of the *Annals of Internal Medicine*. Dr. Sox has served as chair of the U.S. Preventive Services Task Force, the Medicare Coverage Advisory Committee, the Institute of Medicine Committee to Study HIV Transmission Through Blood Products, and the Institute of Medicine Committee on Health Effects of Exposures in the Persian Gulf War. He is a member of the Institute of Medicine of the National Academies. A general internist, Dr. Sox has served as president of the American College of Physicians. Dr. Sox has also served on the editorial boards of several journals, including the *New England Journal of Medicine*. Dr. Sox was the principal author of *Medical Decision Making* (1988), the editor of *Common Diagnostic Tests* (1987), and the editor or author of eight other books. In his research and writing, Dr. Sox has explored issues such as technology assessment, medical decision making, disease prevention and health promotion, cost-effectiveness analysis, physicians' and patients' risk preferences, and medical education.

Allen Daniels, LISW, Ed.D., is professor of clinical psychiatry in the Department of Psychiatry at the University of Cincinnati College of Medicine. He also is the chief executive officer of University Managed Care, which has two operational units: Alliance Behavioral Care, a regional managed behavioral health care organization, and UC HealthPartners, a medical disease management company. All of these organizations are affiliated with the Department of Psychiatry at the University of Cincinnati. Dr. Daniels is active on a number of boards and professional organizations. In 2002 he chaired the American College of Mental Health Administration's Annual Summit on Translating the Institute of Medicine's report *Crossing the Quality Chasm* for behavioral health care. He has participated in two Institute of Medicine committees, the committee on Crossing the Quality Chasm: Priority Areas for Health Care Improvement and the Committee on Crossing the Quality Chasm: Adaptation to Mental Health and Addictive Disorders. Dr. Daniels has published extensively in the areas of managed care and group practice operations, quality improvement and clinical outcomes, and academic health care. He has lectured and consulted both nationally and internationally on these subjects. He is a graduate of the

University of Chicago School of Social Services Administration and the University of Cincinnati.

Kay Dickersin, M.A., Ph.D., is a professor of epidemiology at the Johns Hopkins Bloomberg School of Public Health and currently serves as the director of the Center for Clinical Trials and the director of the United States Cochrane Center (USCC), 1 of 12 regional centers in the international Cochrane Collaboration. The Collaboration aims to help people make well-informed decisions about health by preparing, maintaining, and promoting the accessibility of systematic reviews of available evidence on the benefits and risks of health care. From 1994 to 2005, the USCC coordinated development of the Cochrane Central Register of Controlled Trials, which includes nearly 500,000 controlled trials, most of them published. Dr. Dickersin is a member of the Institute of Medicine (IOM) of the National Academies and she has been a member of numerous IOM and National Research Council committees, including the Committee on Research in Education (2002-2004), the Committee on Reimbursement of Routine Patient Care Costs for Medicare Patients Enrolled in Clinical Trials (1998-1999), the Committee on Defense Women's Health Research (1996-1997), the Forum on Drug Development (1993-1995), and others. Dr. Dickersin received a B.A. and an M.A. in zoology from the University of California at Berkeley and a Ph.D. in epidemiology from the Johns Hopkins University School of Hygiene and Public Health in 1989.

Robert S. Galvin, M.D., is the director of Global Health Care for General Electric (GE). He is in charge of the design and performance of GE's health programs, totaling over $3 billion annually, and oversees the 1 million patient encounters that take place in GE's 220 medical clinics in more than 20 countries. Drawing on his clinical expertise and training in Six Sigma, Dr. Galvin has been an advocate and leader in extending the benefits of this methodology to health care. Dr. Galvin has focused on issues of market-based health policy and financing, with a special interest in quality improvement, payment reform, and the assessment of medical innovations. He is a past member of the Strategic Framework Board of the National Quality Forum. He is currently on the board of the National Committee for Quality Assurance and is a member of the Task Force on the Future of Military Health Care. He is a cofounder of the Leapfrog Group and is the founder of Bridges to Excellence, one of the first pay-for-performance initiatives. Dr. Galvin is widely published on issues affecting the purchaser side of health care, and is professor adjunct of medicine at Yale University, where he directs the seminar series on the private sector for the Robert Wood Johnson Clinical Scholars fellowship. He is a fellow of the American College of Physicians.

Dana P. Goldman, Ph.D., holds the RAND Chair in Health Economics and is director of the Peter Bing Center for Health Economics. He also is an adjunct professor of radiology and health services at the University of California at Los Angeles (UCLA). Dr. Goldman's research combines applied economics with health care delivery; and he has been published in the top medical, economic, statistics, and health policy journals. He is on the editorial boards of several research journals, including *Health Affairs*. The sponsors of his research include the National Institutes of Health, the National Institute on Aging, the National Cancer Institute, the U.S. Department of Labor, the Centers for Medicare & Medicaid Services, the Agency for Healthcare Research and Quality, the National Science Foundation, and the California HealthCare Foundation. Dr. Goldman is a past recipient of the Alice S. Hersh New Investigator Award, which recognizes the contribution of young scholars to the field of health services research. He also received the National Institute for Health Care Management Research and Educational Foundation award for excellence in health policy. Dr. Goldman is a research associate with the National Bureau of Economic Research and Director of the UCLA/RAND Postdoctoral Health Services Research Training Program. He received a Ph.D. in economics from Stanford University and a B.A. summa cum laude in economics from Cornell University.

Richard A. Justman, M.D., is national medical director of UnitedHealthcare, a national health service delivery company. He works in the Clinical Advancement division. Dr. Justman is accountable for medical technology assessment, clinical support of pharmacy programs, and clinical support of benefit administration. He has been with UnitedHealthcare since 1993. Dr. Justman received a B.A. from Cornell University and an M.D. from the State University of New York at Buffalo. He is board certified in pediatrics and received postgraduate training at The University of Chicago Hospitals and Clinics and the Johns Hopkins Hospital. Dr. Justman practiced pediatrics in Minneapolis, Minnesota, for 15 years before joining UnitedHealthcare.

Arthur A. Levin, M.P.H., is director of the Center for Medical Consumers, a New York City-based nonprofit organization committed to informed consumer and patient health care decision making, patient safety, evidence-based, high-quality medicine, and health care system transparency. Mr. Levin was a member of the Institute of Medicine's Committee on the Quality of Health Care that published the reports *To Err Is Human* and *Crossing the Quality Chasm*. He also served on the Institute of Medicine committee that evaluated the federal quality effort in its report *Leadership by Example*. Mr. Levin serves as a consultant consumer expert on risk management for select Food and Drug Administration (FDA) Drug Advisory Committee meetings and for four years served as the consumer representative on the FDA's Drug Safety and Risk Management Advisory Committee. Mr. Levin is a member of the Committee on Performance Measures of the National Committee for Quality Assurance and the National Quality Forum Consensus Standards Approval Committee. Mr. Levin has also served on numerous New York State Department of Health committees and work groups, most recently one that authored successful legislation to provide oversight of office-based surgery. He earned an M.P.H. from the Columbia University School of Public Health and a B.A. in philosophy from Reed College.

Richard E. Marshall, M.D., is the former chief medical officer and a practicing pediatrician at Harvard Vanguard Medical Associates, a multispecialty medical group of 500 physicians serving 300,000 patients at 16 offices in the Boston, Massachusetts, area. He currently leads the group's research efforts. Dr. Marshall is a Phi Beta Kappa graduate of Stanford University. After earning a medical degree from the University of California-San Diego School of Medicine in 1973, he went on to earn an M.S. in nutritional biochemistry at the Massachusetts Institute of Technology. Dr. Marshall was board certified in pediatrics in 1980. He currently serves on the boards of directors of the following community-based organizations: Fenway Community Health, a community health center and research organization in Boston known for its work on HIV care and prevention, and Massachusetts Health Quality Partners, an organization currently focused on the public release of quality and patient care experience data. He is also a member of the Massachusetts Commission on Gay, Lesbian, Bisexual, and Transgender Youth.

Wilhelmine Miller, M.S., Ph.D., is an associate research professor at the George Washington University School of Public Health and Health Services, where her research focuses on value-based coverage policy and interventions to address social and economic disparities in health. Previously she was a senior program officer at the Institute of Medicine, serving as staff director for the committee that authored *Valuing Health for Regulatory Cost-Effectiveness Analysis* and as co-director of a four-year study on the consequences of uninsurance. Dr. Miller has taught political philosophy, ethics, and public policy in the Departments of Philosophy at Georgetown University and Trinity College, Washington, D.C. She received a doctorate in philosophy from Georgetown in 1997. From 1976 to 1989, Dr. Miller served as a policy analyst and social scientist in the U.S. Department of Health and Human Services. She received an M.S. in health policy and management from Harvard University in 1976.

Sally C. Morton, Ph.D., joined RTI in 2005 as vice president for statistics and epidemiology, and leads a unit of 220 statisticians, epidemiologists, psychometricians, and associated scientists and staff. Previously, Dr. Morton was head of the RAND Corporation Statistics Group from 1995 to 2002 and held the RAND Endowed Chair in Statistics from 2000 to 2005. From 1997 to 2005 she was co-director of the Southern California Evidence-based Practice Center funded by the Agency for Healthcare Research and Quality (AHRQ). At the RAND Corporation, she was also principal investigator of the Medicare Stop Smoking Program, co-principal investigator of the AHRQ Patient Safety Program Evaluation Center, and the data and analysis task leader on the HIV Costs and Services Utilization Study. She held a variety of leadership and statistical roles on numerous other health services projects. Her methodological interests include the use of meta-analysis in evidence-based medicine, the sampling of vulnerable populations, and statistical methods for health services research. Dr. Morton was a member of the faculty of the Pardee RAND Graduate School, taught at the University of California-Los Angeles School of Public Health, and was an adjunct professor at the University of Southern California Marshall School of Business. She is an editor of *Statistical Science* and served as an associate editor for the *Journal of the American Statistical Association* and the *Journal of Computational and Graphical Statistics*. She serves on the National Institute of Statistical Sciences Executive Committee and is a member of the Educational Testing Service's Data Advisory Committee for the National Assessment of Educational Progress. She was a member of the National Academy of Sciences panel on small-area estimation of school-age children in poverty. Dr. Morton is president-elect of the American Statistical Association (ASA). She is a fellow of the ASA and of the American Association for the Advancement of Science. She received a Ph.D. in statistics from Stanford University.

Samuel R. Nussbaum, M.D., is executive vice president and chief medical officer for WellPoint, Inc. He oversees corporate medical policy, clinical pharmacy programs, health improvement and quality resources, programs for clinical excellence, disease and care management, and health information technology to optimize care for members. His principal responsibilities include serving as the chief spokesperson on medical issues, guiding the corporate vision regarding quality of care and its measurements, leading efforts to assess cost of care performance and developing a strategy to foster further collaboration with physicians and hospitals to strengthen and improve patient care. Dr. Nussbaum also has responsibility for the Health Management Corporation and HealthCore subsidiaries. Dr. Nussbaum has served as president of the Disease Management Association of America, chairman of the National Committee for Quality Health Care, chair of

America's Health Insurance Plan's (AHIP's) Chief Medical Officer Leadership Council, and a member of the AHIP board. He received the 2004 Physician Executive Award of Excellence from the American College of Physician's *Executives and Modern Physician* magazine. Dr. Nussbaum is a professor of clinical medicine at the Washington University School of Medicine and serves as adjunct professor at the Olin School of Business, Washington University. Dr. Nussbaum served as executive vice president, Medical Affairs and System Integration, of the BJC Health System and is president of its medical group. Dr. Nussbaum earned a medical degree from Mount Sinai School of Medicine. He trained in internal medicine at Stanford University and the Massachusetts General Hospital and in endocrinology and metabolism at Harvard University and the Massachusetts General Hospital, where he directed the Endocrine Clinical Group. His clinical and basic research has led to new therapies for the treatment of skeletal disorders and new technologies for the measurement of hormone levels in blood.

Diana B. Petitti, M.D., M.P.H., is adjunct professor of the Department of Preventive Medicine, University of Southern California Keck School of Medicine. She is also the vice chair of the U.S. Preventive Services Task Force. Dr. Petitti served on the National Cancer Policy Board (1997-2003), including as co-chair, the Board on Population Health and Public Health Practice (1995-1997), and has co-chaired three Institute of Medicine committees (Committee on New Approaches to Early Detection of Breast Cancer: Accelerating the Flow from Concept to Clinic; Committee on Large-Scale Science and Cancer Research; and the Committee on Cancer Survivorship: Improving Care and Quality of Life After Treatment). Dr. Petitti earned an M.D. from Harvard Medical School in 1975. After an internship, she spent two years as an Epidemic Intelligence Service Officer with the Centers for Disease Control and Prevention. She received an M.P.H. from the University of California-Berkeley School of Public Health in 1981 and was board certified in preventive medicine in that year. Dr. Petitti was a member of the Technology Assessment study section of the National Center for Health Services Research from 1983 through 1987. She has authored more than 200 scientific publications. Her book, *Meta-analysis, Decision Analysis, and Cost-effectiveness Analysis: Methods for Quantitative Synthesis in Medicine* is widely used to teach the methods for evidence synthesis in schools of medicine and public health. From 1993 to 2006, while at Kaiser Permanente Southern California, she participated in this organization's activities in technology assessment, performance measurement and quality assessment and improvement while simultaneously holding positions as the director of research and evaluation (1993-2003) and senior advisor on health policy and medicine (2004-2006).

Steven Shak, M.D., is chief medical officer of Genomic Health, Inc., which focuses on improving the quality of treatment decisions for cancer patients. He and his colleagues have worked together with leading oncology clinical research groups in the United States to use new molecular diagnostic methods and rigorous clinical studies to develop the Oncotype DXTM breast cancer assay. Dr. Shak has previously served as senior director and staff clinical scientist at Genentech, Inc. where he led the clinical team that gained approval for trastuzumab (Herceptin®), a targeted biological treatment for metastatic breast cancer. He also initiated the cancer clinical trials of the anti-angiogenesis agent bevacizumab (Avastin®). In addition, Dr. Shak discovered dornase alfa (Pulmozyme®), a mucus-dissolving enzyme that is approved worldwide for the treatment of the genetic disease cystic fibrosis. Dr. Shak also held faculty positions at the New York University School of Medicine and Bellevue Hospital from 1978 to 1986. Throughout his career in academia and industry he has focused not only on the science and medicine of drug, device, and diagnostic development but also on the public health issues of access, cost, and appropriate use of expensive new technologies. Dr. Shak served on the board of an independent, non-profit endowment dedicated to expanding access to Pulmozyme therapy to qualifying uninsured and underinsured cystic fibrosis patients. He also participated in establishing a multicenter epidemiological study of the natural history of cystic fibrosis to describe the practice patterns of cystic fibrosis caregivers and to identify prognostic factors for morbidity and mortality. Dr. Shak has collaborated in drug development with many patient advocacy organizations. He is currently on the board of directors of the Children's Cause for Cancer Advocacy, a pediatric cancer advocacy organization, and the Cystic Fibrosis Foundation. Dr. Shak has received numerous awards and honors for his contributions to medicine and patient care. Dr. Shak has an undergraduate degree from Amherst College, an M.D. from the New York University School of Medicine, and postgraduate training in medicine and research at Bellevue Hospital in New York City and the University of California, San Francisco.

Lisa Simpson, M.B., B.Ch., M.P.H., F.A.A.P., is professor and director of the Child Policy Research Center at Cincinnati Children's Hospital Medical Center and the University of Cincinnati Department of Pediatrics. The Center provides evidence-based information to inform policy and program decisions at the local, state, and national levels with an emphasis on strategies to improve the quality of health care, the effectiveness of public programs, and child well-being. Dr. Simpson, a board-certified pediatrician, is the national director for Child Health Policy at the National Initiative for Children's Healthcare Quality, an education and research organization dedicated solely to improving the quality of health care provided to children, and serves as an elected member on the board of directors of two national professional associations, AcademyHealth and the Ambulatory Pediatric Association. She was formerly the All Children's Hospital Guild Endowed Chair in Child Health Policy and professor of pediatrics, nursing, and public health at the University of South Florida, deputy director of the Agency for Healthcare Research and Quality, and the Maternal and Child Health director in Hawaii. Dr. Simpson earned her undergraduate and medical degrees at Trinity College (Dublin, Ireland) and a master of public health at the University of Hawaii. She has received numerous awards including the Excellence in Public Service Award from the American Academy of Pediatrics, the Senior Executive Service Meritorious Presidential Rank Award, and the U.S. Department of Health and Human Services Secretary's Distinguished Service Award.

Glenn D. Steele, Jr., M.D., Ph.D., became president and chief executive officer of the Geisinger Health System in 2001. In this capacity, he serves as a member of the Geisinger Health System Foundation board of directors, an ex-officio member of all standing committees of the board and chairman of the subsidiary boards. Dr. Steele joined Geisinger from the University of Chicago, where he served as the Richard T. Crane Professor in the Department of Surgery, vice president for medical affairs and dean of the Division of Biological Sciences and the Pritzker School of Medicine. Prior to that he was the William V. McDermott Professor of Surgery at the Harvard University Medical School, chair of the Department of Surgery of New England Deaconess Hospital, and president and chief executive officer of Deaconess Professional Practice Group. Dr. Steele is widely recognized for his investigations into the treatment of primary and metastatic liver cancer and colorectal cancer surgery. He is a past chair of the American Board of Surgery and serves on the editorial boards of numerous prominent medical journals. His laboratory investigations have focused on the cell biology of gastrointestinal cancer and pre-cancer. A prolific writer, he is the author or co-author of more than 450 scientific and professional articles. Dr. Steele is a member of the Institute of Medicine of the National Academies of Sciences and the New England Surgical Society and is a fellow of the American College of Surgeons, the American Surgical Association, the American Society of Clinical Oncology, the Society of Surgical Oncologists, the Commonwealth Fund, Healthcare Executive Network, the U.S. Department of Health and Human Services' National Advisory Committee on Rural Health, and the Center of Corporate Innovation. He serves on the American Hospital Association (AHA) Health Care Systems Governing Council and the AHA Strategic Policy Planning and Hospital/Medical Staff

Committees. Dr. Steele received a B.A. in history from Harvard College and an M.D. from the New York University School of Medicine. He completed an internship and a residency in surgery at the University of Colorado, where he was also a fellow of the American Cancer Society. He earned a Ph.D. degree in microbiology at Lund University in Sweden.

Index

Subpopulations, 8, 59, 61, 93, 94, 96, 105, 138, 166, 199, 200, 202
Substance Abuse and Mental Health Services Administration (SAMHSA), 83, 84
Synthesis of results of studies, 7-8, 45, 49, 82, 104-108, 109, 110, 126-132. *See also* Meta-analyses
Systematic reviews
  analytic framework, 89-95
  appraising evidence, 100-104, 110
  availability of evidence, 93-94
  best-evidence approach, 91, 92, 98
  bias, 7, 8, 91, 97-98, 100, 102, 108, 158, 159
  and clinical practice guideline development, 83, 85, 105, 111, 123, 127, 133, 134
  data extraction errors, 102
  database searches, 98-99, 101
  defined, 3, 24, 82-83
  fundamentals, 14-15, 87-108
  hand searches, 99-100
  hierarchies of evidence, 7, 102-104, 108
  international efforts, 84
  journal standards for reporting, 105-108, 155, 159, 199-203
  language/terminology standards, 7, 9-10, 11, 14, 81, 104, 108, 146, 155-156, 159, 166, 171, 172, 173
  methods, 6-8, 14-15, 81, 85-87, 109, 110, 154, 159
  new and emerging technologies, 6, 111-112, 166
  number annually, 58, 59
  objectivity, 6, 7, 86, 157, 165
  origins, 85-87
  priority setting for, 13-14, 62-63
  producers and users, 43, 46-47, 61, 83-85, 133, 156-157, 186
  public access to, 84, 155
  quality issues, 6-8, 49, 81, 86, 100-104, 108, 123, 127, 134, 153, 154, 159, 165-166
  question formulation, 87-88, 92
  recommendations for, 11, 13-15, 81-82, 108-110, 173
  research workforce, 8, 11, 14-15, 36, 82, 109-110
  resource requirements, 124

searching for evidence, 95-100, 127
selection criteria for studies, 89-92, 110, 127
sources of evidence, 86, 94-95, 98-100
standards, 14, 81, 100, 108, 155-156, 159, 199-203
subscription fees, 84
synthesis of results of studies, 7-8, 45, 49, 82, 104-108, 109, 110, 126-132, 159; *see also* Meta-analyses
transparency, 7, 49-50, 51, 86, 104, 105, 155, 159
updating, 73, 111, 158
value of, 3, 6-8, 82, 83

T

Technology assessments
  defined, 24
  milestones, 25, 26
  priority setting, 6
  producers, 43, 44, 163
Transatlantic Inter-Society Consensus, 65
Transparency
  in guideline development, 11, 50, 121, 125, 126, 139-140, 144, 147
  in systematic reviews, 7, 49-50, 51, 86, 104, 105

U

Union County Health Committee, 65
United Kingdom, national program, 161-163
UnitedHealthcare, 20, 66, 67-68, 189
University of California at Los Angeles, 130
Up-to-Date database, 47
U.S. Breastfeeding Committee, 65
U.S. Department of Defense, 42, 163
U.S. Department of Health and Human Services (HHS), 9, 10, 61, 153, 164, 171, 172
U.S. Food and Drug Administration (FDA), 26, 42-43, 50, 51, 64, 83, 84, 93, 112, 131, 143, 207, 216, 218
U.S. Office of Technology Assessment (OTA), 26, 27